# baby

## COMES HOME

Library and Archives Canada Cataloguing in Publication

Roumeliotis, Paul, 1957-, author
Baby comes home : a parent's guide to a healthy and well first 18 months / Dr. Paul Roumeliotis M.D.

Includes bibliographical references and index.
Issued in print and electronic formats.
ISBN 978-1-77141-072-4 (pbk.).--ISBN 978-1-77141-076-2 (html)

1. Infants--Health and hygiene. 2. Infants--Care. I. Title.

RJ101.R69 2014 618.92 C2014-905887-X
C2014-905888-8

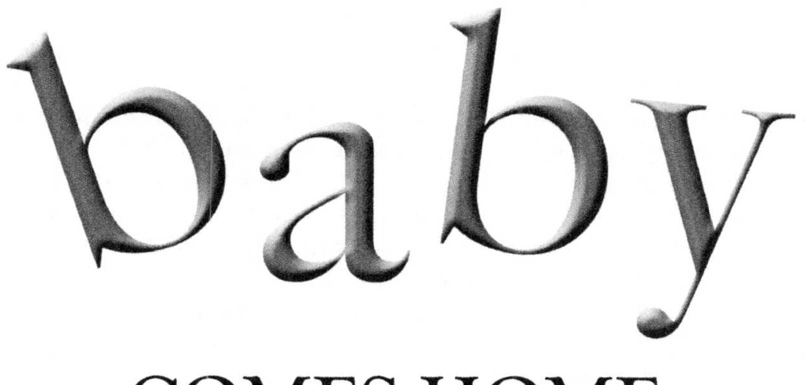


# COMES HOME

A Parent's Guide to a Healthy and Well
First Eighteen Months



Dr. Paul Roumeliotis, M.D. CM, MPH, FRCP(C)

First Published in Canada 2014 by Influence Publishing



Book Cover Design: Marla Thompson
Editor: Nina Shoroplova
Typeset: Greg Salisbury
Author Portrait Photographer: Jean-Marc Carisse

This book is dedicated to the loving memory of my father, Petros Roumeliotis. He was a great man and an even better dad.

# TESTIMONIALS

*"Dr. Paul, an expert in pediatrics, has written a groundbreaking book about the importance of childhood/infant health in preventing illness and ensuring wellness later on in life. An accessible and valuable resource for doctors, psychiatrists, paramedics and parents around the world, this book should be used by organizations to further global initiatives relating to pediatric health on the international stage, the main specialized bodies of the United Nations, UNICEF and WHO in particular. If you are one of the believers of my own quote on this very subject: "A sound mind can only be found in a sound body," then I strongly recommend that you carefully read and digest this innovative book by Dr. Paul accordingly."*

**His Excellency, Ambassador Doctor Waheed Waheedullah, United Nations Chief Trouble Shooter, Mother Theresa Peace Prize Winner**

*""Baby Comes Home" highlights how important the first few months of a baby's life are. From delving into the science of the developing brain to exploring the daily routines of infant care, Dr. Paul has written an informative and engaging book about ways to invest in your baby's current and lifelong health and wellness. I wish Dr. Paul's book had been around when my five kids were growing up! He has anticipated the questions parents have and gives answers in a clear no nonsense way. He even makes the science understandable. This will be a well-thumbed book by all new parents and frequent late night reading!"*

**Dr. Jean Clinton, MD, FRCP(C), Infant and Child Psychiatrist & Assistant Clinical Professor, Psychiatry and Behavioural Neuroscience, McMaster University**

# ACKNOWLEDGEMENTS

I would like to first and foremost acknowledge the unwavering support of my wife Diana, my daughter Helen, and my son Peter. It was only through their understanding and patient encouragement that I was able to complete this book. I also wish to thank my parents for the sacrifice they made to immigrate to Canada over half a century ago that offered me an otherwise unattainable opportunity to obtain a first-rate education and pursue my passions and aspirations.

During my more than thirty years in the medical field, I have had the privilege of training and working with countless exceptional physicians and teachers, many of whom are world leaders and pioneers in their respective fields. However there are three colleagues in particular that I would like to recognize, who collectively have influenced my career journey that ultimately led to the conceptualization, preparation, and completion of this book.

Dr. Jean Clinton, Associate Professor at McMaster University and member of the Offord Centre for Child Studies, is a renowned infant and child psychiatrist who inspired me to focus this book on the first eighteen months. I have the pleasure of working with her presently, as she is a true champion for early child development and support. Her devotion and strong advocacy for the provision of a loving, caring, and nurturing environment to babies is indeed contagious. She continually reminds her audience, be it politicians, decision makers, or health professionals, that a baby's brain needs to be continually stimulated in order to develop to its full potential. I admire her ability to passionately communicate this information and I attribute a lot of what I wrote about in the first part of the book to her teachings.

Between 1986 and 1987, I had the privilege of spending most of my final year as a pediatric resident at the Montreal Children's Hospital working with Dr. Ron Barr, who is currently Professor of Pediatrics, University of British Columbia and Head, Developmental

Neurosciences & Child Health, Child and Family Research Institute at the BC Children's Hospital. As my mentor, he taught me a tremendous amount about developmental and behavioural pediatrics. Equally importantly, by observing his interactions with parents and colleagues, I learned about the value of compassion and kindness in pediatric practice that he demonstrated so well. Serendipitously, now decades later, I have the pleasure to work with Dr. Barr once again in raising awareness about his work on infant crying patterns and the prevention of Shaken Baby Syndrome.

Dr. Nicolas Steinmetz, former Executive Director of the Montreal Children's Hospital is the third colleague that I would like to mention. When I became an attending staff at the Montreal Children's Hospital, he provided me unequivocal support as I established the hospital's outpatient Asthma Program in 1990, one of the first of its kind in North America. The Asthma Centre re-grouped a then novel, dedicated multidisciplinary team that formally embedded parent/patient education into the treatment protocol. The success of this pioneering approach was proof of my belief that that the more parents know, the more comfortable they are with their children's health and wellness. This experience also reinforced to me the vital role of communication and education in the everyday practice of medicine. In addition, Dr. Steinmetz was one of the very few colleagues who understood and recognized the relevance of my health communications vision, back when digital media and the internet were in their infancy.

I would also like to recognize and thank the expert team at Influence Publishing: Julie Salisbury, publisher, Nina Shoroplova, editor, Alina Wilson, Gulnar Patel, Greg Salisbury, Lyda McLallen, and Trista Baldwin. Their input, cooperation, and support was invaluable in the creation of the final version of this book.

Finally, this section would not be complete if I did not mention my love for kids, our future leaders, and for music, a major driving force that motivated and shaped my career path.

# CONTENTS

# Welcome and Introduction by Dr. Paul

Congratulations on your new arrival! Becoming a parent is one of the most exciting and rewarding experiences in life. Many first-time, and even experienced, parents may admit that they're unsure about how to properly care for and ensure the health and wellness of their new baby. I firmly believe that the more you know about what to expect from your newborn, the more comfortable you will be. This is why I coined the phrase: "When it comes to your child's health and wellness, Knowledge Is Comfort."

It is also comforting to understand exactly what your rapidly developing newborn needs to ensure that he or she will grow as well as possible. I have dedicated most of my career to creating and distributing and sharing child health and wellness information to parents and child caregivers worldwide, and I am delighted that I now can finally present some of my work in this, my first formally published book.

In this reference guide, I describe what parents and child caregivers can do to ensure that baby is well-nourished, healthy and well, free from injury, and growing in a nurturing environment. Specifically, I will review the newborn baby period from the moment of birth and offer basic and important baby care and safety information through to your first eighteen months together and beyond. This includes addressing frequent parental concerns and describing some of the most common illnesses and conditions seen during the first few years of life. Much of what I write can be thought about and done before baby comes home. For example, preparing your new baby's room, making sure that you have a properly installed car seat to bring baby home in, finding a healthcare provider, and babyproofing your home (both indoors and outdoors).

This book is a collection of knowledge and information drawn from my clinical practice and teaching experiences, readings, and my publications and productions. Specifically, I have tried to address the most common questions of parents and caregivers since I started working in the field of pediatrics in the early 1980s and launched my website (www.drpaul.com), as the world's first on-line pediatrician, in 1995. I have selected and compiled the material for this book from the hundreds of articles and fact sheets that I have created for newspapers, magazines, videos, radio, and the internet. Constantly updated and reviewed, the information I present or adapt, represents currently accepted best practice guidance and knowledge. You will notice that I place a heavy emphasis on prevention. This reflects that, since 2007, my career has shifted toward a broader public health practice, yet with a focus on child health and wellness, recognizing that the best start possible will ensure a long, healthy, and prosperous life.

When I was putting this book together, one of my major challenges was to determine the sequence of the many topics that I cover. The order of the sections (in the print version) reflect the timing and frequency of questions from parents of newborns, combined with topics that I think are important to know about as early as you can. Specifically, I include injury prevention early on, although I do not typically get many questions about this from new parents. Where possible, within each section, I list the chapter titles and headings in alphabetical order for ease of use. There are several ways this handbook can be used. You can read the whole book from the beginning to end ahead of time, and refer back to any topic as needed. Or you can use it as a handy reference guide by skipping to specific sections or chapters as the need arises.

As I live, work, and trained in North America, for many topics, I adapt or refer to positions, guidelines, and recommendations from relevant recognized organizations based either in Canada or in the US. Most of the time, these recommendations are generally similar and thus applicable to both countries. If there is ever a difference between Canadian and American approaches, I will point them out. Despite my "North American" origin, much of the knowledge that I share is relevant worldwide, especially when it comes to what children need during their first few years of life.

Although the title says *A Parent's Guide*, this book can be a helpful resource for any child caregiver, be it a grandparent, aunt or uncle, babysitter or daycare teacher. In addition, many of the topics that I cover will apply even beyond the age of eighteen months. I also want to remind you that the information provided in this book is meant to be an educational aid only. It is not intended to replace the advice and care of your healthcare professional, nor is it intended to be used for medical diagnosis or treatment. If you suspect that your child has a medical condition, always seek medical attention. Please note that any mention of specific brand names or products in this book is only for educational purposes and is not meant to be an endorsement of any kind.

## Why Are The First Eighteen Months So Important?

Most books about newborn babies concentrate on handling and feeding, or are mostly about physically caring for a new baby. Uniquely, I take an additional approach, because we now understand from advances in neurobiology, neurophysiology, and gene studies that what happens early on in life can have consequences many decades down the road. Although children of all ages have special and specific needs to grow and develop normally, the first eighteen months of life are crucial. In fact, "the first twenty-seven months" would be a more accurate description, because the nine months of pregnancy are equally important. For the purposes of this book, I will concentrate mostly on the extremely important and formative first eighteen months of a baby's life.

I have written this book with a huge emphasis on ensuring that baby is safe, and grows and develops normally. In simple terms, I describe the ideal conditions for a baby to live and grow in. These include proper nutrition, injury prevention, immunization, and of course, very importantly, the provision of tender loving care. I look at this as a guide to wellness, starting in the first eighteen months and lasting a lifetime.

### The Early Years Are So Important: The Science of Tender Loving Care

Science has now shown that responding to your baby's needs, caressing, touching, and stimulating baby are very important interactions … from day one of life. Why is this so? As a baby develops, many changes in the brain related to such vital functions as language, learning, emotional regulation, social ability, vision, and perception occur at a very fast pace. Most of this complicated development is well underway by eighteen months of age. It all relates to the baby's brain growth, also known as sculpting. More specifically, babies are born with many more brain cells (neurons) than adults and the ones that get used are the ones that remain. During the first few years of life, these brain cells start to develop connections that on the outside we see as development. When the baby's brain grows, it is actually these nerves—the wiring—that are forming, interconnecting, and expanding. From a practical point of view, when we measure and chart a baby's head size, we see that most of its growth occurs during this period. In fact, the head size—the head circumference—of a twenty-four-month-old baby is almost 80 percent of the size of an adult's head.

So it is important during this period of growth that babies are in a situation and environment that promotes (allows) their brains, nerve cells, connections, and learning/cognitive abilities to develop to their full potential. We know that, if they do not achieve this development properly or fully, there can be long-term consequences. These effects may not be obvious early on in life, but may appear years or even decades later.

Obviously, as parents, we want our babies to grow and develop as normally as possible in order to reach their full potential as adults. In this regard, parents and other caregivers can do some very simple things to help ensure that their baby develops as normally as possible. Soothing your baby when he or she is upset is one of the most important things you can do. Babies learn to regulate or control their emotions by first being soothed by you. Reading to baby, making eye contact, caressing, playing with baby, and giving baby loving attention are things that are very inexpensive and quite easy to do, virtually anywhere, anytime, and under any circumstances. For example, the relatively new practice of skin-to-skin contact at birth has been shown to help this development and nerve-connection formation.

I urge you to discover and connect with your new baby. Look into your baby's eyes, smile, and glow! In response, baby will smile back and his or her brain will receive these signals to positively promote and foster the vital sculpting and wiring process. By establishing and maintaining this relationship with new and growing babies, you can help them develop to their full potential. I would prescribe this approach from the very first minute of birth, to be done by everyone caring for baby.

## Looking Into Baby's Future ... And Being Able To Shape It Positively!

This concept of being able to shape a baby's future positively has been examined very closely recently. In fact, there is a new term: "Life Course Perspective." This recognizes that experiences early in a baby's life build connections that have effects on development—emotional and physical growth— that can have lifelong behavioural and even physical consequences. We know that genes play a role in determining one's potential and characteristics. This relatively new field of study is known as epigenetics. Epigenetic research clearly shows that negative and positive external or social environmental factors can modify how and when genes get turned on or off. This modification actually affects one's genetic potential or programming. When this happens repeatedly, it is known in the scientific world as biological embedding; where the gene, more specifically the DNA actions, can be changed by external surroundings. This modification can result in abnormal development of a gene's role that may or may not be immediately obvious or visible. This is also true during pregnancy. Of course, proper nutrition, injury prevention, and immunization remain vitally important; but now we know that, in addition, attention needs to be paid to ensure that babies are soothed, stimulated, caressed, and nurtured as much as possible. TLC—tender loving care—is not a new concept; we always suspected it was important, and now we have the science to prove it.

The Life Course Perspective explains how early experiences in life can impact long-term health and functional capacity. We have long known that effects of certain insults and stressors to a developing child are visible and obvious. For example, the use of the medication thalidomide in the 1960s to ease a mother's morning sickness during pregnancy is an example of inadvertent drug damage that resulted in very visible consequences with babies born with missing limbs. The genes and DNA required to form normal limbs were "epigenetically" silenced by the medication so the limbs did not grow. However, there are many other types of damage and consequences that are not immediately apparent, but which may add up over time to create significant negative effects. What is also new is that we now know that this just doesn't happen during pregnancy. These negative effects include social disadvantage, abuse, neglect, a lack of bonding (a lack of TLC), environmental insults, and more. From the point of view of the baby's brain, these are referred to as outside sources of toxic stress, which can have very negative and even permanent effects on a baby's brain development and ultimately on overall emotional and physical well-being.

For example, decades ago, babies born small for gestational age (low birth weight) were thought to simply catch up and grow normally without any long-term problems. These babies were seemingly full term, looked and behaved normally, but had lower than average weights at birth. Now, studies have shown that these babies (referred to as IUGR, for Intra Uterine Growth Retardation), as adults, have higher rates of diabetes, high cholesterol, and heart disease as compared with babies born with average birth weights. This means that our genes can somehow be modified or affected by the environment. In this case, by the uterus, perhaps due to malnutrition or other factors. This demonstrates the importance of prenatal care during pregnancy.

We also know that physical and emotional stress or abuse can result in long-term health effects. For example, people who are persistently prejudiced against have higher rates of chronic disease than those who do not face discrimination of any kind.

Here is another example of the effects of neglect on physical health and well-being: I have seen babies admitted to hospital with growth failure who almost miraculously, once admitted, started to gain weight. This is because the nurses and other hospital staff that took care of them showed affection and care. Sadly, these babies came from home situations of neglect or even abuse. This was my first exposure to the physical effects of neglect or abuse on young babies.

Studies on the effect of brain and hormone controls by the lack of bonding, healthy relationships, and nurturing during the first few year of life have shown rather worrisome results. Animal studies, and to some extent human studies, have proven that lack of maternal care, stimulation, and love (affection) results in abnormalities in the Hypothalamic-Pituitary-Axis (HPA). The HPA is a series of brain, nerve, and hormonal system connections that control the secretion of important hormones including adrenaline and cortisol. These hormones are referred to as stress hormones. Studies have confirmed that HPA damage or misdevelopment can be caused by neglect, even during the first few months of life, resulting in hormonal imbalances that can last decades, and by accumulating damage, can actually cause chronic medical disease. This relates to the brain sculpting and wiring period I described earlier in this section. Up until now, it was very clear that lack of bonding and nurturing in babies can result in long-term psychological and mental conditions. It is now also clear that this neglect can exacerbate or even cause chronic physical illness such as diabetes and metabolic syndrome even decades later. So, investing in a child's early support not only assures proper mental, emotional, and psychological development at the time, but indeed is a form of chronic disease prevention.

A study by the University of Toronto reported that adults who were abused as children had a higher risk of heart disease as compared to adults who were not abused as kids. This finding, once again, highlights the importance of the role of a nurturing environment for both a child's present and future life. Babies need to be loved, cuddled, and stimulated in order to grow and develop normally. When they are sick, afraid, stressed, or unhappy, babies and young children need to be soothed by caring adults in their life. Infants and children who are abused or neglected are robbed of this effect and indeed end up with higher rates of both mental and physical illness in the future. Today we know that neglect has more significant effects on a baby's development than physical abuse. The aspects of a child's development that are interfered with play a role in a child's future learning and socializing skills, and ultimately their ability to reach their full potential as adults.

School readiness and ability to socialize and interact are also dependent on early year support and nurturing. In North America, there is a clear correlation between developmental maturation as measured through the Early Development Index (EDI) and the family's socioeconomic profile. In general, the poorer and more disadvantaged children are, the less ready for school they are, as compared to children from richer and less deprived social environments. Once kids enter school already behind their peers, they tend to remain behind and can never catch up. Sadly, the consequences and multiple effects can last a lifetime. These include dropping out of school, poor employment prospects, poverty, social isolation, and chronic medical illness. However poor parents who read to their children and, give them lots of TLC can actually protect their kids from this disadvantage.

## TLC is Free!

Now, let's look at all this in a positive way! Regardless of your home, family situation, or environment, it does not cost anything to respond to, nurture, caress, and give your baby as much attention as you can.

The back and forth interaction of smiles, gurgles, and eye contact with babies literally builds their brains! Connecting and interacting with baby and establishing a relationship are easy to do and the pleasure you will get back is priceless. At the same time, baby's brain is feverishly developing and growing well. Playing peek-a-boo and other games and activities that stimulate your baby, which I discuss in a later section, is easy, affordable, and portable. Even talking to your baby about anything will be helpful. Actually, the more face-to-face words a baby is exposed to, the better will be the vocabulary at three years of age, and this translates into better success in reading and other related academic activities in grade school. All of this to say that baby's emotional and physical development and growth really rely on the environment and the social connections and relationships that a baby is exposed to.

It is reassuring to know that despite growing up in poor environments, children have become healthy, prosperous, and successful adults. Why? As babies, they received attention and TLC from the many members of the immediate and extended families they lived with. They were passed around among all the relatives living together, be they siblings, grandparents, uncles, aunts, or family friends. This attention from the surrounding family is really a community of relationships and connections. Not surprisingly, communal TLC and attention promote normal (even optimal) brain development, which later in life means overall wellness and success. All this in poor or disadvantaged conditions from the material point of view. The opposite is true too. Being born into a rich family situation, does not guarantee normal development and future prosperity and wellness. Even in rich families, if the parents are too busy or preoccupied with other things and do not provide the necessary attention, stimulation, and TLC, their babies too may end up with negative future mental, emotional, and/or physical consequences. Once again, infant-parent and infant-caregiver relationships and connections do not cost anything; yet, there is so much return!

## Technical Aspects of Stimulating Your Baby

As I have described, a baby's brain needs to receive stimulation in order for it to grow to its full potential. For instance, a baby needs to be able to hear for speech to develop. From a technical point of view, the following types of stimuli are needed:

- Sound;
- Vision;
- Smell;
- Touch;
- Proprioception (sensing one's own body movements and position); and
- Taste.

Any interaction with a baby involving these senses will stimulate the complicated nerve connection and wiring growth process of the baby's brain. If there is no stimulus or input, that part of the brain will not fully develop or grow properly. In fact, babies who have been subject to extreme neglect, at three years of age, have smaller brain sizes than babies who grow normally. Dr. Jean Clinton, a renowned infant and child psychiatrist and colleague, puts it very simply: "If you don't use it, you lose it." In other words, if the brain cells do not get stimulated they will not develop, grow, and connect as they should. Practically, all of these forms of stimulation can be easily achieved by establishing a relationship with baby right from the moment of birth. More specifically, breastfeeding provides all of the above sensations and stimulations. However, anyone caring for baby can help. This is all in an effort to help support the brain's neuron connection formation and organization, which will positively influence the child's future mental, emotional, and physical development!

## Reading: A Concrete Example of What Parents Can Do

I want to discuss reading to baby as one easy thing that parents can start right after birth. There are many benefits to reading to our children.

### Language and Speech Development

Reading to a child makes it easier for him/her to develop speech. As a matter of fact, I recommend that parents read to children who have speech delays as part of their treatment.

### Vocabulary

The number of spoken words babies are exposed to influences how large their vocabulary will be by age three. The more you read and talk to your baby, the more words baby hears and stores.

### Preparing for School

Children are ready to go to school when they can attend or listen to what someone else is saying, in this case, the teacher. Reading to a child is a great way to prepare for learning and participating in a structured school environment.

### Bonding Time

Reading to a child is also an ideal opportunity for a parent to spend some time with their child. Reading time can be perceived as "our time!" Needless to say, this is an easily built-in opportunity to cuddle and nurture baby!

### Part of a Routine

Reading to children before bedtime becomes a nice pre-bedtime ritual or routine. Children tend to have an easier time going to sleep if there is a set routine.

### Life-Long Benefits

As children get older, they will read on their own, building on the interest and experience of being read to for years. This sets off a life-long interest in reading, which comes in handy in many aspects of our lives.

After reading this section, I hope you agree that the "Best Beginning Possible" is important for all babies. Such a good start not only means providing for a child's physical needs, but also for creating and fostering a safe, loving, and nurturing home and family environment. This is the best investment in a child's future that parents, child caregivers, and society as a whole can make. I hope that this book helps you ensure the best possible future for your precious new baby!

## Before Baby Comes Home

If you have other children, one important part of baby's arrival home is to prepare them for the arrival of their new baby brother or sister. Younger children may feel threatened by the new baby, and these concerns should be addressed before baby arrives. If you already have children, involve them. You don't want them to worry that they're being left behind. So to help prevent later problems like sibling rivalry, reassure your children that they are loved, and involve them in preparations for the baby's arrival. The more they are involved, the more they will feel part of your growing family. It may be a good idea to have a small gift prepared so you can give it to them as a gift from the new baby. New babies typically receive a lot of gifts (not to mention attention), so a young child may be jealous—receiving a nice gift from the new baby is a great way to offset jealous feelings and a great way for the older brother or sister to meet the new baby!

## At the Hospital

Soon after delivery, your baby's weight, length, and head circumference are measured. These measurements are very important as they will be used in the future for comparing and assessing your baby's health and rate of growth. A doctor will also quickly examine your baby to make sure that everything is okay.

The baby's eyes are then treated with silver nitrate eye drops or antibiotic ointment to help prevent infection. She'll also be given an injection of vitamin K to help the clotting ability of her blood.

A small amount of blood will be taken from the baby's heel to be tested for a number of conditions. It will also be used to test for your baby's blood type. Within twenty-four hours, the baby is weighed again, and given a more thorough examination. You may wish to be present for this exam, as it's a good time to ask the doctor any questions.

Healthy full term babies are usually sent home from the hospital or birthing centre within twenty-four to forty-eight hours of birth, or longer if they were born via C-Section. Should there be any problems, if the baby was born prematurely, or if it was a multiple birth, the stay will be longer, depending on the individual situation.

### Baby's First Physical Examination

The first physical examination of your newborn is extremely important to ensure that your baby is screened for any problems or congenital anomalies and is healthy. Many elements of the examination, including how a baby looks, moves, and behaves, the shape of the head, the positioning and shape of the eyes and ears can be important clues.

Here is a head-to-toe summary of what the newborn physical examination involves.

- The head and face are examined to ensure there are no bumps, bruises, or swelling. The fontanels (soft spots) are also felt and the head circumference is measured and recorded. A light is shone into the eyes to ensure that there are no cataracts or other eye defects. The ears, nose, mouth, and tongue are also examined, with particular attention paid to the palate and lips. The examiner will also test for the presence of the suck reflex. When a finger is placed in their mouths, newborns normally (instinctively) begin to suck. The neck is assessed for any bumps and to ensure that it can turn easily both ways, right and left.
- The chest and abdomen are inspected for any obvious abnormalities. The heart and lungs are evaluated by feeling the precordium area (the centre of the chest) and by listening (auscultating) with a stethoscope. The examiner will also feel for pulses in the arm, groin, and foot areas, and may also need to measure the blood pressure of the upper and lower limbs. The abdomen is examined by feeling (palpating) for any abnormalities and listening with a stethoscope.
- The genital and groin areas are assessed for any abnormalities or bumps (hernias). In boys, the scrotum is examined to ensure that both testicles are present and there are no other problems.
- The nervous system is generally assessed during the whole exam by how a baby reacts and how stiff or soft the muscles are (assessing muscle tone). The reflexes are tested with a small reflex hammer. The baby is also examined to ensure that the startle reflex (the Moro reflex) is present. With your baby lying on his or her back, the examiner gently pulls up and holds baby slightly off the table by the arms and then suddenly releases. This sudden release

causes the typical startle reaction, which is a jittery shaking of all four limbs for a few seconds. This can also be seen at home when babies are startled by a loud noise or sudden movement. All normal newborns have the Moro reflex; it disappears within the first few months of life.

- The skin on the entire body is inspected for any rashes, birthmarks, or similar problems.
- The spine (from the neck to the buttocks area), clavicles (collarbones), arms, and legs are examined with particular attention to the hips. The fingers and toes are also carefully assessed and counted.

# Taking Baby Home

## Car Seats, Car Safety, and Passenger Air Bags

Before taking your newborn home from the hospital, make sure you already have a government-approved infant car seat professionally (properly) installed in your car. The car seat should be placed so that the infant is facing backwards. All infants and toddlers should ride in a rear-facing car seat until at least the age of two years, or until they reach the highest weight or height allowed by the car seat's manufacturer. Until the baby is strong enough to support his or her own head, the car seat should have special liners or a rolled-up blanket wrapped around baby's neck to support her head. Infants and children under age twelve should never sit in the front passenger seat of cars equipped with air bags, even if he or she is in a car seat. The explosive impact from a deployed passenger side air bag can seriously injure a child.

To repeat, when installing a car seat for the first time, make sure that this is done as per the manufacturer's instructions and make sure it fits well into your car. Not all car seats fit all models of cars. Also read the section on car seats in your car's owner manual; it may help you ensure that the installation is done properly. It is important to keep the car seat instructions, as you will need them to adjust the seat as your baby grows. Once properly adjusted, your child's seat harness should be snug, but not too tight; you should be able to fit the width of two fingers between the child and the harness. The buckle should be chest-high.

Contact the manufacturer to ensure that there are no recalls of the model you purchased. It is also useful to fill out and send in your registration card to the manufacturer, as it will be important in case your car seat is recalled. A new car seat is more likely to meet the current standards and be of a far better design than most second-hand or hand-me-down seats—especially those more than two-years old. Older car seats are unlikely to adhere to today's safety requirements. Also, a lot of people do not realize if the car seat has been in a car crash, and looks right, it may have been weakened, and therefore should not be used.

Use the car seat at all times while out driving. Never try holding your child in your arms. During rapid braking at just thirty miles per hour, a ten-pound baby in your arms will seem to weigh more than two hundred pounds and you won't be able to hold on. Believe me, I have seen the tragic consequences of children injured in car accidents while sitting on their parents' laps. Using a properly sized, installed, and adjusted car seat **every** time you take your child for a ride is certainly your best bet.

Parents often ask which brand or make of car seats is the best. There really is no one seat that is the best or safest. The best car seat is the one that fits your baby's size and weight, and can be correctly installed in your car. So it would be important to try before you buy. If possible, put your child in it to see if it is the proper size and make sure it fits into your car.

It is important to know that an improperly installed or an unsafe car seat can result in severe injury in case of an accident. For more specific information, visit the American Academy of Pediatrics article on "Car Seats: Information for Families for 2014" at: www.healthychildren.org/English/safety-prevention/on-the-go/Pages/Car-Safety-Seats-Information-for-Families.aspx.

# Baby's New Home Environment

## Baby's Environment

Babies are sensitive to extremes of temperatures, so keep the home comfortably warm, but not hot or cold. During winter, don't place a heavy blanket in your baby's bed for added warmth, because heavy bedding poses the risk of suffocation. Instead, turn up the room's thermostat to a more comfortable temperature. The baby's room should always be kept between or 20° to 22° Celsius or 68° to 72° Fahrenheit, with humidity at around 40 percent. During hot summer weather, an air conditioner may be used to keep the room at this temperature if necessary.

## Avoid Crowds

A baby's immune system—their defense system—is not fully developed at birth and so they are more susceptible to infections. For this reason, it is recommended that babies less than three months of age not be brought into places with large crowds or gatherings such as malls, restaurants, etcetera.

Also, it's very important to keep your baby's environment smoke-free. Exposure to second-hand tobacco smoke increases a baby's risk of developing asthma, ear infections, and a host of other medical problems. Indoor air pollution, more than outdoor air pollution, causes and/or worsens respiratory disorders in children, especially in those with sensitive airways. Second-hand smoke, kerosene space heaters, and improperly installed wood stoves produce odourless, yet potentially harmful, combustion products in high concentrations in the household.

## Second-Hand Tobacco Smoke Avoidance

Small children who passively breathe in cigarette smoke are at a higher risk for getting ear infections, colds, pneumonia, and asthma. In addition, environmental tobacco smoke can cause other symptoms including a stuffy nose, headache, loss of appetite, and fussiness. So don't smoke or allow others to smoke in your home and in confined spaces such as the car.

During my years working with children who had asthma, I was struck by the number of kids who reported that their parents or guardians smoked at home. So my personal feeling from this experience was that there is a link between asthma and second-hand smoke exposure. Of course, this impression is supported by the many scientific studies that have proven the negative effect of second-hand smoke on children.

Here are some facts that I think will explain why health experts are so concerned about the effects of second-hand smoke, especially for children:

- One puff of tobacco smoke contains hundreds of dangerous chemicals, some of which are known to cause cancer. Actually, when one smokes, the filter in the cigarette itself may partially block some of these products from being inhaled. However, when one is inhaling passive smoke from another smoker, there is no filter. Children are especially susceptible to second-hand smoke, because, for the same level of exposure, they will absorb more of these toxins than adults do due to their small size.
- Children exposed to environmental tobacco smoke have increased rates of lower respiratory tract illness and increased rates of ear infections, asthma, and Sudden Infant Death Syndrome (SIDS, also known as crib death). Also, it is well known that a

child's developing respiratory system is more susceptible to infections and toxins during the first few years of life as compared to adults. Tragically, exposure during childhood to environmental tobacco smoke may also be associated with development of cancer during adulthood.

- Recent studies have also shown that third-hand smoke, for example going into a room where someone had smoked previously, is also a potential danger. Many people are surprised to find out that many of the toxic chemicals found in tobacco smoke do not have an odour.
- Babies born to mothers who were exposed to second-hand tobacco smoke during pregnancy have been shown to have nicotine and other tobacco-related chemicals in their urine after birth. To be clear, the mothers did not actively smoke during pregnancy; they were exposed to second-hand smoke, and still, traces of the toxins were found in their newborn babies' urine.
- Of course, if a mother smokes during pregnancy, the baby is directly exposed to these toxins and it is well known that among other problems, babies born to mothers who smoke are smaller than normal at birth, and tend to have higher risks of asthma and other respiratory conditions.
- Second-hand smoke in vehicles is more concentrated than in most other circumstances, and can be up to twenty-seven times greater than in a smoker's home.

The above facts are very convincing. By protecting our loved ones, especially our children from second-hand smoke, we help them toward living as healthy and well a life as possible.

# Keeping Baby Safe: Injury Prevention

This section will review the potential dangers and sources of injury as well as what precautions parents and caregivers can take to prevent injury both at home and outside the home. The single greatest threat to your child's health comes in fact from injuries, especially at home and in the car. Indeed, accidental injuries are the leading cause of hospitalization and, tragically, death in children in North America. The good news is that most injuries are preventable. This is why I chose to present this section early on in my book. I believe that you should be thinking about injury prevention, and identify and address some of the risks to your baby even before your newborn comes home. Once baby arrives, you will probably have very little time left to think about injury prevention. Instead, you will be preoccupied by the basic baby care issues such as getting to know new routines, feeding needs and patterns, all of which I address in subsequent sections of my book. By taking a few simple steps ahead of time, you can greatly reduce your baby's risk of injury and better guard your child's precious health. Prevention is best! A good place to start is at home where most childhood injuries occur. The first step to babyproofing your home is to get down on the ground to get a child's view of things. Look for anything that may be dangerous and remove it from reach.

# Home Safety

## Baby's Room

### Furniture and Crib Safety

Look for a baby mattress with holes that allow air to circulate, to prevent suffocation. Firm mattresses are next safest, to prevent the risk of suffocation. Avoid a soft mattress. For the same reason, pillows should not be placed in the crib for the first year. As well, to prevent the risk of strangulation, the crib's bars should be no further than two and a quarter inches or about 5.5 centimetres apart. When covering or wrapping baby in sheets and blankets, be sure he or she can breathe easily.

All children's furniture, especially cribs, should meet the most current government standards. Older cribs with railings too wide apart are at least as dangerous as having no railings at all, since the child could become trapped between them. So look for furniture that meets current standards and minimizes the child's chances of injury. When buying a crib or bed, look for places where a little head or limbs could be pinched or trapped—for instance between a mattress and its frame, or between crib bars.

Once a child is old enough to stand, keep out of their crib toys like activity centres and any toy that can be used as a step. Toys have been known to act as a helping step out of the crib and onto the floor—often headfirst.

### Rocking Cradles

Rocking cradles can be great for soothing a child, but they shouldn't be used once the child can push herself up on her arms, or is able to roll over, which can be as early as three months. By this early stage, she could easily topple herself over. Keep a rocker on the ground, never on a table, bed, or dresser. If the baby falls asleep in the rocker, put wedges under the legs to stop further rocking. No matter what, never leave a child unattended in a rocker.

### Diaper Changing Tables

Falls from a changing table are not uncommon, so they should have effective guardrails or raised edges. Have all the supplies you need at hand so that you won't have to leave the baby unattended, even for a few moments.

### Infant Carriers

A hard plastic type infant carrier seat placed on a counter-top, table, washer/dryer, etcetera is another common cause of serious falls among infants. Therefore, always place infant carriers on the ground.

### Chairs and High Chairs

If you don't have a high chair, prevent falls by restraining the child in his or her seat with something like a scarf tied around the waist, under the arms, and around the back of the chair. Never prop up a young child in an adult chair, regardless of whether you use pillows or not. Babies left on their own can easily topple over, often headfirst.

### Shelves, TV Stands, and Wall Units

Be careful with TVs as children have been injured by pulling a TV set down onto themselves from freestanding TV wall units and stands. Also, be aware that children have been injured trying to climb wall unit shelves, so take the necessary precautions to prevent this.

### Toy Safety

Be careful of toys with small button batteries. These tiny batteries can be swallowed by young children. Button batteries can be toxic and dangerous if swallowed. If you suspect that your child has swallowed one, seek medical attention immediately.

## Bathroom Safety

Bathtub and toilet drownings are quite common. So always pay full attention to your child in the bath. Have everything you need for bath time close at hand, and don't leave your child in order to answer the phone or the door—even while the bath is just filling. It's not worth the risk.

To avoid injuries and drownings from bathtub falls, use a slip-resistant mat or decals. Also, discourage your children from standing in the bathtub.

Keep toilet lids closed at all times. Better yet, install and use toilet lid latches.

At all times, keep all medications, vitamins, cosmetics, and personal care items safely out of reach and locked away in the medicine cabinet or cupboard. Also, be sure to keep cleaning products and other chemicals locked away and out of your child's reach. To further help prevent poisonings, install and always use child-resistant cupboard locks and drawer latches.

Always use properly sealed child-resistant packages for all medications, even for vitamins. Also, bear in mind that many child poisonings from medication, vitamins, and minerals happen at grandparents' homes and other such places where child-resistant packaging is not customarily used.

## Being Prepared for Emergencies

Part of taking care of baby is ensuring that your family is prepared for an emergency situation. Emergencies can occur at any time and can take many shapes and forms. Natural emergencies include flooding, earthquakes, illness outbreaks or pandemics, ice storms, severe thunderstorms, tornados, hurricanes, and heat waves. There can also be man-made emergencies, such as air and rail accidents, transport vehicle accidents, industrial accidents, and terrorist attacks.

Some emergencies occur suddenly without warning, while others may have warning signs beforehand. One thing that all major emergencies have in common is that they can potentially disrupt our normal daily activities, cause damage to property and the environment, and in some cases may even threaten our lives and those of our loved ones.

Governments at all levels have developed their own emergency preparedness plans, which include a review of local potential hazards or risks and preparation of response plans for a variety of emergencies. This involves the coordination of many people, many departments, and many levels of government, starting from municipal to county to the provincial or state level. However, the main point is that emergency preparedness begins at home. It is important for you to have your own emergency plan and a survival kit ready at all times in case of an emergency that would require you to leave your home or be without power and the other amenities of your home.

For everybody's sake, it is worth all the time and planning in order to be as prepared as possible. When preparing your home and family for an emergency, make sure you hazard-proof your home, keep emergency numbers handy (including the closest hospital, municipality, and utilities), and prepare a survival kit. As your baby gets older or if you have older children, it is a good idea to teach them what the number 911 is for and how and when to dial it. An emergency survival kit should contain enough of the following items to keep you and your family self-sufficient for at least three days.

An emergency survival kit should contain these items:

- Water;
- Non-perishable food;
- Flashlight;
- Crank radio or battery-operated radio with spare batteries;

- Blankets and sleeping bags (one per person including blankets for your young children or babies);
- First aid kit;
- Candles and matches or lighter;
- Extra car keys and cash;
- Important papers (identification card for everyone, personal documents);
- Clothing and footwear;
- Toilet paper and other personal supplies;
- Medication;
- Whistle;
- Playing cards and games.

All these items should be stored in a bag that you can take with you. Remember to review your emergency kit on a regular basis, and try not to use its contents except during an emergency. Events such as ice storms and severe storms and flooding are examples of what can happen. For the near future, experts are predicting very unstable and extreme weather as a result of global warming. So now is a good time to prepare if you have not already done so. It is worth the time and energy for the peace of mind of knowing that you and your family are ready for any emergency.

## Burn and Fire Prevention

### Burn and Scald Safety

Most accidental burns in young children are scalds due to accidents in the kitchen, so do not hold baby while also handling a hot drink. If you must, be sure the drink is at the most only warm, never steaming. Spilled hot tea or coffee could seriously burn your baby.

Coffee pots and teapots or any other containers full of hot liquids or food should not be kept or left on the table if you have toddlers in the home. Always make sure that the handles of the pots and pans are facing the back of the stove and use the rear elements if possible.

One of the most common bathroom injuries comes from scalding hot tap water. Always run bath water and test the water temperature yourself before the child gets in. Besides these measures, set the maximum temperature on your hot water tank to 48° C (110° F). Check the water temperature before putting children in a bathtub. The safest temperature for bathing is about 37° C (100° F).

Also, be aware that electric baseboards, radiators, and vents from hot air furnaces can get really hot. Make sure these are screened with guards or that your young child does not have easy access to these potential sources of burn injury.

Young children should not be allowed to play near hot ovens, barbeques, or other sources of heat.

Parents of small children should use a cool mist humidifier when necessary instead of a steam vaporizer or humidifier

Also, never leave a child unattended around the stove, oven, or microwave in the kitchen

## Fire Safety

Most serious injuries in the home are caused by house fires and falls. Household fires cause about 75 percent of all deaths related to fires and burns; so, prevention is best!

Here are some tips and facts on fire and burn safety.

- Smoke detectors save lives. There should be at least one on each floor of your home, and more if possible, especially in children's rooms. Smoke detectors should be regularly tested and always have fresh batteries. It's one of the least expensive yet best investments you can make for your family

- Don't smoke in bed. The leading cause of house fires where a child has died is smoking in bed.
- Work out an action plan with the whole family about what you will all do in case of a fire. Plan and practise alternative escape routes from every room in your home.
- You should own and know how to use at least one all-purpose fire extinguisher. Be sure your extinguisher is always fully charged and regularly inspected by a trained technician.
- If you have disposable lighters in the house, make sure they are child-resistant. Always store matches safely out of the reach of children.
- Check and secure all potential sources of heat and burn injury. Place screens on fireplaces, woodstoves, and kerosene heaters.
- Clothing that you dress your children in should be flame-resistant or flame-retardant. This means that these cloths have been treated with special chemicals that prevent or resist flames.

## Choking Prevention

Babies and young children can choke on virtually any object. Tragically, children have died from choking on things such as small balls, tiny toys, balloons, and plants. According to Safe Kids Worldwide, almost sixty percent of choking incidents were food-related. Thirteen percent of cases involved swallowing coins and nineteen percent involved candy or gum. A recent study released by the American Academy of Pediatrics (July 2013) found that more than twelve thousand young children per year are brought to the emergency room for choking. Many of these children choked on food. In 1997, more than half of all choking deaths in children were related to latex balloons. We tend to think of balloons as fun objects, but we should be aware of their potential for tragedy.

- When visiting other people's homes, remember that their homes may not be childproofed. When arriving at a party or friend's house, look around to make sure that there are no obvious hazards for your child.
- When going out to holiday parties without the children, be sure that your babysitter knows where and how to reach you. All emergency numbers should be clearly posted, so that the babysitter can use them if needed.
- To avoid food poisoning, always thaw the turkey in the refrigerator and not on the countertop. Also, remember that food should never be left at room temperature for more than two hours, as it will spoil. Spoiled foods are covered by invisible, yet potentially dangerous germs that cause food poisoning.
- Children love to get toys for Christmas! It is a good idea to follow the age ranges on toy packaging, as toys that are too advanced could be hazardous for younger children. Make sure that there are no parts of the toy that could be swallowed or could choke a child.
- Small children enjoy stuffed toys like Teddy bears and cloth dolls. When buying these items, make sure that they have sturdy seams and that the eyes, noses, and other parts are very firmly attached. Loose pieces can easily be swallowed by a child.
- Make sure that your young child does not have access to the Christmas tree. Ornaments are often made of metal, plastic, or foam, and can be dangerous as they can block the child's air passage and can also cut a child's skin.
- Holiday plants are quite attractive to children, but potentially very toxic. Make sure that plants such as Mistletoe, Holly, and Rhododendron are out of reach of children at all times.
- Giftwrapping paper often contains toxic metals and, therefore, children should not be allowed to chew it. Additionally, do not

burn giftwrapping paper in the fireplace as it may give off toxic fumes.

- Toy ideas for children less than one year old include wooden blocks, floatable toys, squeeze toys, and soft animals without buttons or other parts. Do not give babies small toys that can be swallowed, or toys with long strings that may potentially strangle a child.
- Toy ideas for the over-two-year-old include developmental toys that encourage the imagination to expand. Projectile-type toys such as guns, weapons, and toys with sharp edges or points are inappropriate.

## Easter Safety

Here are some Easter safety suggestions.

- Be sure that Easter toys and dolls (such as bunnies, chicks, etcetera) are free of choking hazards. Pieces that can be removed from a doll or toy pose a potential choking danger to small children.
- In order to prevent choking, do not give small candies or chocolates to children less than five years of age.
- Chocolate Bunnies are an Easter tradition. However, be very careful when giving such gifts to children who are allergic to peanuts or nuts. Make sure you read the label of contents, as many chocolates, although said to be "pure chocolate," may have been in contact with nuts or peanuts during the preparation and packaging processes.
- Eggs are potentially hazardous foods, in the same category as meat, poultry, fish, and milk. In other words, they are capable of supporting the rapid growth of disease-causing bacteria like Salmonella . Before boiling eggs for Easter decorating and painting, they must be kept refrigerated.
- Never leave raw eggs in any form at room temperature for more

than two hours. Don't eat or cook with cracked eggs or eggs that have been unrefrigerated for more than two hours.

- Hard-boiled Easter (decorated) eggs left at room temperature for many hours or days as a decoration or table centrepiece should be discarded and not eaten.
- Use only clean, unbroken eggs. Discard dirty or broken eggs. When you boil your eggs, make sure the water is hot 85° to 90° C (185° to 190° F). Cool your eggs in cold water or just in the air.
- Cleanliness of hands, utensils, and work surfaces is essential in preventing the spread of bacteria. Always wash your hands when handling eggs, especially between cooking, cooling, and dyeing. Wash hands again, along with all utensils, equipment, and counter tops that have been in contact with any raw food before preparing other foods.

## Halloween Safety

Do your best to make Halloween safe. Thinking about safety in advance will make all the difference! Here are some tips that can help your child have a safe Halloween.

### Costume Safety

- Halloween costumes and accessories should be safe and should not be flammable (they should be flame-repellent). Also, make sure that the costume is not so long that the child could easily trip on it.
- Do not allow your child to wear high-heeled shoes as they can cause a child to trip more easily.
- Avoid dark Halloween costumes as your young trick-or-treaters need to be fully visible in the dark. Bright costumes are better.
- Carrying fluorescent bags, wearing glow-in-the-dark stickers,

and reflective material or tape will help make your child more visible in the dark. Bringing along a flashlight is helpful, too.

- Halloween masks can prevent a child from seeing well and this can be quite dangerous, especially at night when it is dark to begin with. Creative, non-toxic makeup is safer.
- When your child is carrying costume accessories such as a plastic sword or fork, make sure that the accessories are made of soft plastic, bend easily, and are not dangerously sharp.

**Making Your Home Safe for Trick-or-Treaters**

- To keep your home safe for visiting trick-or-treaters, remove anything a child could trip over such as garden hoses, toys, bikes, and lawn decorations.
- Check that the outdoor lights work and replace burned-out bulbs if necessary.
- Wet leaves can be quite slippery, so they should be swept away from sidewalks and steps.
- Remind all neighbourhood drivers to remain cautious and drive slowly throughout the community.
- Don't leave your pets outside at Halloween, as they can either get accidentally injured or they may attack one of the children who are trick-or-treating at your door.

**Pumpkins and Other Decorations**

- Do not overload electrical outlets with holiday lighting or special effects.
- Small children should never carve pumpkins. Children can draw a face with markers, then parents can do the cutting. Under parental supervision, children ages five to ten can carve with

pumpkin cutters equipped with safety bars.

- Lighted pumpkins should be placed on sturdy surfaces, away from curtains and other flammable objects.
- Halloween candles inside Jack-O-Lanterns, for instance, should not be left lit at home unattended while you are out trick-or-treating with your young ones. Battery-powered lights can safely do the trick instead.
- Make sure that Jack-O-Lanterns with candles in them on the porch are far enough away from children, so they won't accidentally trip on them and their costumes won't be accidentally set on fire.

**Treats**

Try to portion out treats for the days following Halloween.

- Although sharing is encouraged, make sure items that can cause choking (such as hard candies) are given only to those of an appropriate age.
- Parents with children who have food allergies should be extra careful that their kids do not eat any of the treats until they've been checked.
- Also, never leave your child's loot bag unattended.
- Remember to instruct your children not to eat any of the Halloween treats they collect before an adult has inspected them. If anything is not wrapped, looks suspicious, torn, opened, or tampered with, throw it away. Eat homemade treats only if you know the giver.

### When Trick-or-Treating

As your baby grows older or if you have older children, the following tips will be helpful while you go out trick or treating:

- Plan and review with your children the route that is acceptable to you. Have them remain on well-lit streets, always use the sidewalk, and agree on a specific time to return home.
- Trick-or-treaters should use a flashlight (with fresh batteries), so that they can see and be seen by others. They also should never cut across yards or road shoulders, and always remember to walk and never run across a street.
- Children should be accompanied by an adult and only visit familiar homes. They should be instructed to never enter a house they are trick-or-treating at, and to avoid dark or deserted-looking homes.
- Teach your children to stay away from strangers, to refuse to approach or climb inside cars, and to stay away from stray animals.
- Teach your children to be careful of moving cars and obey traffic lights, to stay on one side of the street at a time, and when that side of the street is finished, then carefully to cross and trick-or-treat on the other side. Children should not be crisscrossing a street back and forth.

## Kitchen Safety

Do not hold baby while you cook, or while reaching for something on your upper shelves. Instead, put him or her in a playpen, or on a play mat on the floor near a wall, ideally in a corner. It's a lot less trouble if baby has his or her own regular, out-of-the-way spot, where everyone in the house knows to expect him or her to be.

Many children are poisoned by ingesting household chemical

products. It is customary for us to keep cleaning supplies, etcetera, below the sink. But get into the habit of keeping these products on upper shelves, completely out of the reach of children.

When shopping, look for products that come in child-resistant packages. Don't leave sharp objects unattended. Sharp dangers even include small things like plastic bread bag hooks and wire twist ties, which should be kept in a safe place or put in the garbage so they don't fall into the wrong hands.

Don't leave anything hot unattended. Make a habit of turning pot handles away from the edge of the stove, counter-top, or table.

Toothpicks, common items not thought of as a source of danger, can actually cause injury. It is estimated that there are more than eight thousand toothpick-related injuries per year in the US. Most occur to the eye and ear. Toothpicks should therefore be kept out of the reach of babies and young children.

## Other Home Safety Precautions

### Safety Around Windows

Open windows, even with screens can be dangerous. Young children can fall from screened windows and can be quite seriously hurt or even die from their injuries. Screens are not a strong protection against falls and they give a false sense of security. Here are some tips to prevent falls from windows:

- Use window guards that create a barrier, or window stops that limit the amount the window can open. Windows should not be able to open more than four inches.
- Do not put any furniture or any other objects in front of a window; children can climb these to get to the window.

### Blind Cord Safety

Low hanging blind cords can potentially strangle a baby and young child. To prevent strangulation from blind cords,

- Supervise your baby and young child at all times.
- Tie-up blind and drapery cords or cut them so they are out of the reach of children.
- Never leave loops hanging.
- Do not place cribs, dressers and other pieces of furniture near windows to prevent your child from climbing and getting tangled in blind cords that are left hanging.

### Stairs and Falls

Falling down stairs can often result in serious head injuries, so it's very important to properly install stair gates at the top and bottom of all stairways. Also, do not use baby-walkers on wheels, as their use has resulted in severe injuries from falling down stairs while in these walkers. Never leave your child unattended on a table or other high place, even for just a few seconds as they can roll off in the blink of an eye.

## Pet Safety

Many children are bitten by animals, mostly domestic pets. When a new baby arrives into a home setting with a pet accustomed to being without children, the pet may be jealous. The parent cannot assume the pet is safe around the newly arrived child. Never leave your new baby alone with your pet. If necessary, have your pet kept in a kennel or a friend's home and be very careful when the pet first sees your new baby.

Another related problem is that pet food is a potential danger for babies, especially when they start crawling and exploring by putting everything within their reach into their mouths. Aside from being a choking hazard, pet food has been the cause of bacterial outbreaks including *Salmonella* in children less than two. These children had eaten their home pet's tainted dry pellets or chunks.

Here are some precautions to take to protect your baby and young children, if you have pets at home.

- Wash your hands after touching pet food and bowls;
- Regularly clean feeding bowls and the area where they are placed;
- Pick up the pet bowls from the floor when they are not in use;
- Keep babies and young children away from the pet food and the pet bowls;
- Do not clean pet bowls in the kitchen sink; use the bathroom sink or the tub.

## Protecting Your Family Against Rabies

The rabies virus infects the central nervous system (the brain and spinal cord), and is found in mammals, mostly raccoons, foxes, and especially bats. However, rabies can affect domestic pets, as well. This is why vaccinating pet dogs and cats against rabies is important.

### How Does Rabies Infect Humans?

The rabies virus is found in an infected animal's saliva and can be transmitted through bites or contact of the animal's saliva with eyes, mouth, or an open wound. In humans, if the virus enters the body and spreads, it is usually fatal, as there is no effective treatment for an active rabies infection. However, there are vaccines and specific serum injections that are given on a precautionary basis if a person has been bitten by a potentially rabid animal. These injections are known as Post Exposure Prophylaxis (PEP) injections. The incubation period—the time between getting bitten and developing rabies—is not clear, but it can be at least several weeks or longer.

## Preventing Rabies

The following will help protect your family and your pets from rabies:

- Have your cats and dogs vaccinated.
- Do not feed wild animals.
- Teach children to stay away from wild or stray animals.
- Take measures to discourage wild animals from taking up residence in your home or on your property.
- Do not attempt to trap wild animals that are causing damage to your property. Contact a professional animal control officer, instead.
- Report any animals behaving strangely to your local animal control office or municipality.
- Do not touch dead or sick animals.
- Do not nurse sick animals.
- Have all dead, sick, or captured bats that have come into contact with a human or pet tested for rabies. Do not touch the bat. Contact your local health authority or agency for details.

### What to do for Animal Bites

- A person may need to receive PEP to prevent rabies if they have been bitten or have been in direct contact with a potentially rabid animal. Local public health authorities are notified of all animal bites and will proceed with the following:
  - Obtain details of the circumstances of the bite.
  - Obtain details about the animal's overall state including vaccination proof for domestic animals.
  - If the biting animal (cat or dog) is available, alive, and well, it will be isolated and observed for ten days. If during this period, the animal shows signs of rabies, PEP will be administered to the bite victim.

- If the animal is available in the case of wild animal bites, it will be sent for testing. If it tests positive for rabies, the victim will be administered PEP.
- If the biting animal (either wild or domestic/stray) is not available, then health authorities may offer PEP as a precaution.

Note that each situation is unique and handled based on the individual circumstances including the type of animal, the context of the bite, and the local rabies incidence data.

## Plant Safety

Parents are surprised to find out that some of the most common poisons ingested by children come from plants. Therefore, all plants in the home should be identified, in order to know whether or not they are potentially toxic. Additionally, plants and related parts should be kept away from young children. The following plants are poisonous if ingested:

- Dieffenbachia;
- Jerusalem cherry;
- Mistletoe;
- Holly;
- Rhododendron.

### Important Facts and Tips About Plant Safety

- All plants in the home should be identified in order to know whether or not they are potentially toxic.
- Plants and related parts including bulbs and seeds should be kept away from young children.
- Move all potentially dangerous plants to a safe place.
- Children should learn at an early age not to drink out of flowers or make tea with leaves, seeds, or berries.

- Do not use unknown plants or trees in making playthings or toys for children.

### Non-Toxic Plants

- African violet;
- Begonias;
- Coleus;
- Dracaena;
- Ferns;
- Jade plant;
- Prayer plant;
- Rubber plant;
- Schefflera;
- Spider plant;
- Swedish ivy.

Know your local Poison Control Centre or emergency room number. If a child ingests a plant, make sure you know the exact name of the plant. It is helpful in trying to find out if it is poisonous and whether or not treatment is needed (if any). Also, take a piece of the ingested plant with you to the emergency room

Keep on hand syrup of ipecac, which induces vomiting. Do not induce vomiting unless you are instructed to do so because, for some poisons, it is dangerous to make a child vomit. Follow your poison control centre or emergency room's instructions.

## Poison Prevention

The five most common accidental ingestions or poisonings in children less than five years of age are:

- Medications, including aspirin, acetaminophen, and vitamins;

- Household cleaners;
- Plants;
- Cosmetics; and
- Pesticides.

Keeping these items and other potentially dangerous substances out of your child's reach is the best protection against accidental poisonings. To prevent poisoning and cuts from sharp objects, install cupboard and drawer latches, especially in the kitchen and bathroom. Toxic substances and medications should **always** be stored high up and away from reach, as should anything sharp.

Many children are poisoned each year by ingesting toxic substances at home. The key is to prevent accidental poison ingestions before they happen. There are hundreds of potentially poisonous products in the average home.

### Here Are Some Tips to Prevent Accidental Poisoning

- Keep in mind that child-resistant packaging is not necessarily fully childproof, as some children, as they get older, can figure out how to open them.
- Always keep medications, household cleaning products, cosmetics, and other potentially toxic substances in locked cabinets.
- Keep purses and wallets in a safe place out of the reach of children.
- Always read the labels on all medication and household product containers.
- Keep all the products in their original containers to be able to identify them in case of accidental ingestion.
- In order to avoid temptation, keep all medications and other potentially toxic substances far out of the sight (and reach) of children.

- Clean out your medicine cabinet regularly and safely discard any expired, unnecessary, or unused medication.
- Never tell children that medicine tastes like candy and avoid taking medication in front of children as they imitate adults.
- When working with toxic or potentially dangerous chemicals, avoid all distractions. If you must interrupt your work (say to answer the phone or the door), make sure first that the containers are closed properly and the area you are working in cannot be accessed by young children.
- Many car owners give their car a tune up, including changing the anti-freeze, oil, etcetera, at home. Be sure that these highly toxic products are always out of the reach of your children.

### Be Prepared in Case of Accidental Poison Ingestion

- Know the local emergency room or poison control centre phone number so that you can contact them for advice immediately.
- Keep on hand syrup of ipecac, which induces vomiting. Do not induce vomiting unless you are instructed to do so because, for some poisons, it is dangerous to make a child vomit. Follow your poison control centre or emergency room's instructions.
- Take the container of the ingested product  or medication with you to the emergency room.

## Safe Sleep Environment

As most parents know, there are plenty of opinions out there on the best way to put your baby down for naps or bedtime. But the safest method for putting your baby down to sleep is more than just a matter of personal preference. Research has shown that some methods carry serious risks, including accidental injury, suffocation, or SIDS. However, you can lower these risks by making sure your baby has a safe sleep environment.

Experts on child health and sudden infant death agree that the safest place for a baby to sleep during the first six months of life is on his or her back, in a crib in your room (which should be smoke-free). Having your baby close to you will make night-time breastfeeding easier, and may help reduce the risk for SIDS. It's also safer than having your baby in bed with you, since bed-sharing has been shown to increase the risk of suffocation and SIDS.

Below are Current Sleep Safety Recommendations for a safe sleeping environment for infants.

### Don't Bed-Share

Sharing an adult bed, sofa, or other soft sleeping surface with your baby increases the risk of SIDS. Your baby is also at risk of becoming trapped, smothered, or suffocated.

### Use a Crib

Place your baby to sleep in your room, in a crib, cradle, or bassinet that meets current applicable safety regulations. Your baby's mattress should be firm, flat, and fit snugly in the frame. Strollers, swings, bouncers, and car seats are not intended for sleeping infants.

### Place Your Baby on His or Her Back To Sleep

While babies should spend some supervised time every day on their tummies to help them develop their neck muscles, at naptime and bedtime, they should be put on their backs.

### Keep Soft Materials out of Your Baby's Crib

Don't use sleep positioners, or place bumper pads, comforters, stuffed animals, pillows, or other items in your baby's crib or bassinet.

### Make Sure Your Baby's Room Is Not Too Warm

Dress your baby in light sleepwear that's comfortable at room temperature. If a blanket is needed, use only a thin, lightweight, and breathable one.

### Keep Your Baby Away From Tobacco Smoke

Make your baby's room and your house smoke-free, and choose a non-smoking caregiver. Don't allow anyone to smoke around your baby.

## Used Toys and Equipment—A Word of Caution

Yard and garage sales are quite popular especially during the spring and summer months. Children's items are popular products at garage sales and yard sales. However, older items may not be safe as they might not meet current safety regulations. These items include the following.

### Used Car Seats

Experts currently do not recommend buying used car seats, as they usually do not come with instructions, and it is essential that car seats are installed and used properly and as directed. If the seat is over ten-years old, it is considered unsafe, in part, because plastic components deteriorate over time. Are all the parts in perfect working order? Is it the right size and fit for your child?

NOTE: A seat that has been in a collision must not be used again. Buyers cannot tell how old the seat is or what has happened to it. All car seats must meet **current** safety standards and carry a compliance label on the side, rear, or bottom of the seat, stating the size of the child for whom the seat is designed. Instructions must be provided on how the seat is to be installed.

### Used Cribs

Cribs made before September 1986 don't meet current safety standards. The mattress support in them—suspended by hooks—is not secure and can collapse easily. These cribs cannot be fixed to meet the standard and must not be sold or given away.

### Used Strollers

Strollers manufactured before 1985 may not meet current standards. Choose one that is both sturdy and safe. The stroller must match the size and age of the child and be sturdy enough to support the child and not be easily tipped.

### Walkers

**Walkers are very dangerous. Expert authorities recommend against the use of baby walkers.**

### Playpens

In 1976, newer playpen regulations were released. Mesh playpens must be made of mosquito-type netting with small holes so that fingers and little buttons cannot get through. Current standards also prohibit the use of more than two castors or wheels on a playpen, to prevent it from moving around too much.

### Baby Barriers and Gates

Since 1990, new regulations have made expansion gates safer. Accordion-style baby gates that are made of wood or hard plastic and have diamond and V-shaped openings and large Vs at the top can no longer be sold. Children can get caught in the openings and potentially strangle or injure themselves.

### Toys

Toys are subject to vigorous safety testing before being allowed to be sold. But not all older toys found in garage sales meet these standards. Also, be logical—toys that are in poor condition, damaged, or broken are clearly unsafe. Lawn darts with elongated tips are dangerous and can no longer be sold.

### Used Electrical Appliances

The greatest risks in buying used electrical appliances are that you do not know how old they are, what abuse they have taken, or the condition of the appliance's electrical components. If you buy a used appliance, make sure it meets your country's current standards. You should also have the product checked by a qualified repair shop before using it.

### Bottom Line on Buying Second-Hand

Garage and yard sales may offer great deals ... but getting something potentially dangerous to you, your family, and others is not worth the savings.

## Vision Health and Safety

Every year, worldwide, millions of people seek medical attention for an eye injury. Our sight is precious yet we tend to take it for granted, especially when our newborn arrives, when eyesight and vision protection are sometimes not obvious priorities. But it's a good idea to think about protecting baby's eyes and vision as part of the routine prevention checklist.

The approach to eye health especially in young children is screening and prevention. Here are some tips to help protect your eyes and your children's eyes at home:

- Point spray nozzles away from anyone's face.
- Use grease shields on frying pans.
- Turn your face away when uncorking bottles.
- Clear rocks and stones off the lawn before mowing.
- Trim low-hanging branches in your yard.
- Avoid toys with sharp edges or points and projectile toys (missiles, arrows, etcetera).
- Make sure toys are not damaged or have any loose or broken parts and are age appropriate.

The biggest threat to our vision health outside the home—aside from accidental injury—is the sun. Long-term exposure to UV light rays increases the chances later on in life of developing cataracts (blurred and clouded vision) and Acute Macular Degeneration, which is a leading cause of blindness. So it is important that you and your children wear sunglasses year-round when outdoors during the day. The glasses should be large enough to protect the entire eye against 99 percent of UVA and UVB rays.

## Water Safety/Drowning Prevention in the Home

Each year, approximately 140,000 people die worldwide from drowning. In the United States, 20 percent of all cases occur in bathtubs. Bathtub drownings most often occur to children who were unsupervised at the time of the accident. Toilet drownings are also quite common. In fact, a child can drown in just a few inches of water. So always pay full attention to your child in the bathroom.

### Other Drowning Hazards at Home

Other than pools, baths, and toilet bowls, there are other water hazards found near or in your home. These include the following:

- Ditches or large puddles of water;
- Postholes;
- Wells;
- Fish ponds;
- Fountains;
- Pails; and
- Any other object that can accumulate water.

Parents and child caretakers should be aware that these pose drowning threats to young, unattended children and they need to watch their children closely if playing near any of these areas.

# Keeping Baby Safe Outside the Home

## Cold Weather Safety Precautions

Winter can be lots of fun, but, unfortunately, there are some associated potential dangers. Once again, young babies are especially vulnerable to extreme cold temperatures and conditions. Here are some facts and important tips about keeping babies and young children safe during the winter.

- Children can easily succumb to frostbite, so during cold weather make sure that your child's clothing, shoes, boots, and gloves stay dry. If any of these items gets wet, change your child into dry ones.
- Make sure your children do not play in snow that is piled up for clearing on the street or sidewalks. Tragically, children have been killed by snow cleaning equipment while playing in these banks.
- As the winter ice and snow melts, it may fall from a roof or the side of a house or building and injure someone seriously. Make sure that your home or building is free from causing this hazard.
- Whenever allowing your children to sled or toboggan, never allow them to slide on or into a road. Additionally, they should go down shallow slopes free of obstacles such as trees and avoid sliding down a crowded slope.
- Most winter sports injuries involve twists, sprains, and strains. These injuries can be prevented, for example during skiing and skating, by getting your child good instructors, proper equipment, and of course appropriate supervision.
- Helmets have become part of the standard equipment and attire

in biking, hockey, inline skating, baseball, and football, to name a few sports. They should also become a regular habit in winter sports or activities that can potentially cause life-threatening head injuries, such as tobogganing and skiing.

- Snowmobiling is particularly risky for children and young adults. For safety reasons, children less than six years of age should never ride as passengers on snowmobiles. Also, only children older than sixteen years of age may drive snowmobiles. Of course, drivers and passengers should always wear the proper protective equipment, including approved helmets.
- Frozen ponds and lakes make for great skating. Make sure, however, that the ice is thick enough to allow safe skating before you let your children walk onto or skate on such frozen surfaces.
- Fireplaces are fun, warm, and cozy, but should be used safely. Always use a screen to prevent sparks from igniting items around the fireplace such as newspapers, carpets, furniture, and curtains. Only use the fireplace when you're at home and awake.
- Install carbon monoxide detectors in your home if your heating system uses fuels such as oil or gas.
- Never leave children in a running parked car, especially during the winter, because the snow can block the car's exhaust pipe, resulting in carbon monoxide poisoning, which can be deadly.

## What Is Frostbite?

Exposure to cold temperature without adequate protection can result in frostbite. The term "frostbite" means that a part of a body has been frozen; this can be quite dangerous. Usually, it is the face, nose, ears, fingers, and toes that get frostbitten. Frostbite can occur during any outdoor activity including play, and especially during fast-moving sports such as skating, skiing, snowboarding, and tobogganing. Obviously, the colder and windier it is, the quicker an unprotected part of the body will become frostbitten. The skin around a frostbitten area initially becomes red, then it pales and, very rarely, it becomes bluish. As the skin warms up there can be some blisters which may be painful.

### Tips on how to Prevent Frostbite

- Children should be dressed warmly with properly fitting clothing. Several thin layers will help keep children dry as well as warm. Clothing should include long johns, turtlenecks, one or two shirts, pants, sweater, coat or jacket, warm socks, boots, gloves or mittens, and a hat.
- Do not let children stay out in the cold too long. Set reasonable time limits on outdoor play; this of course will depend on how cold it is.
- Call children inside periodically to warm up.
- When possible, avoid taking infants and young children outdoors when it is colder than 4° C (or 40° F).
- Use common sense: for example, if there is a cold or frostbite warning issued, do not let your children go outdoors at all.
- Make sure your children's clothing stays dry. Change them into dry clothing immediately, as wet clothing can make frostbite occur more quickly.
- Keep these tips in mind, even for older children and teach them how to prevent frostbite too.

### What Are the Signs of Frostbite?

The signs and symptoms of frostbite include:

- Numbness or pain in the fingers, toes, nose, cheeks, or ears.
- The skin is blistered, hard to the touch, or shiny.

### How Is Frostbite Treated?

Although prevention of frostbite is the best approach, if there is a possibility that your child has frostbite, take the following steps:

- Take the child indoors immediately.
- Call your doctor or local health help line.
- Ask the child to gently move the affected body part to increase the blood supply to that area.
- Warm the white frozen part(s) against the body. Hold fingers to the chest or under the armpits, for example.
- Soak frozen part(s) or area in warm water (not hot water).
- Be gentle, as frozen tissue can damage easily. Do not rub or break blisters and do not massage the frozen area or rub it with snow or ice.
- Frostbite is usually painful. For associated pain, acetaminophen may be needed, administered according to age and weight.
- If the frostbitten area does not improve, remains white, or turns blue, seek medical attention.

## Heat Injury Prevention

### How Does Heat Affect the Body?

Generally, humans can control their internal temperature in the heat by sweating. However, under extreme heat and humidity conditions the body cannot keep up and will suffer from heat stress. The elderly and young children, as well as those with chronic respiratory and heart conditions, are more susceptible to heat-induced injury. Babies under one year of age are extremely sensitive to the ambient temperature. Their body temperature control is not yet mature and their temperature tends to reflect the ambient level. So special care needs to be taken with babies during hot spells.

The effect of heat on the body is a result of three factors: the humidity level, which causes 70 percent of heat stress; sun radiation, which causes 20 percent of heat stress; and the temperature itself, which causes 10 percent of heat stress. It is, therefore, important to understand that the humidity level plays the most important role in heat-induced stress and illness. During heat waves, the temperature is measured, but the humidity is also recorded and tends to bring up the temperature. This measurement is referred to as the "humidex," a term that is short for humidity index.

### About Humidex

The humidex chart below determines when people might wish to take precautions to prevent heat-related illnesses.

| Humidex | Degree of Comfort |
|---|---|
| 20—29 | No discomfort |
| 30—39 | Some discomfort |
| 40—45 | Great discomfort: avoid exertion |
| 46 and over | Dangerous; high risk of heat stroke |

Source: Environment Canada and Health Canada

### General Recommendations for High Humidex Ratings

- Humidex of 35 to 39: Certain types of outdoor exercise should be toned down or modified, depending on the age and health of the individual, their physical shape, the type of clothes they are wearing, and other weather conditions.
- Humidex of 40 and over, which is extremely high: All unnecessary activity should be limited.

## What Are the Consequences of Heat Exposure?

### Heat Exhaustion

Heat exhaustion usually occurs after prolonged exposure to heat and/or heavy exercise in the heat resulting in increased loss of body fluids through heavy sweating. The signs of heat exhaustion include:

- Clammy, pale skin;
- Sweating;
- Dry mouth;
- Tiredness and fatigue;
- Headache; and
- Dizziness.

### How is Heat Exhaustion Treated?

Children suffering from heat exhaustion need to be removed from the heat immediately, given water to drink, and have cool compresses applied to their skin. Fortunately, heat exhaustion is not life-threatening, and will resolve with rest, fluids, and cooling down.

### Heat Stroke

Heat stroke is a very dangerous and potentially life-threatening form of heat stress or injury. The body is so overwhelmed by the heat and humidity that it loses the capacity to sweat. This results in a very high body temperature, which in severe cases can actually cause brain damage and, tragically, even lead to death. Heat stroke can occur suddenly and is an emergency requiring immediate medical attention.

The signs of heat stroke include:

- Very high body temperature—39.5° C (103° F) or higher;
- Hot, red, and dry skin;
- Absence of sweating;
- Deep or shallow breathing;
- A weak pulse rate;
- Confusion or hallucinations;
- Seizures;
- Loss of consciousness.

## Heat Injury Prevention

Clearly, the best approach to prevent heat injury is to limit activity during high humidex times, as heat injury can potentially result in heat stroke, which is very dangerous. Here are some ways to prevent heat injury during high humidity heat waves:

- Young children and babies should be dressed very lightly and not bundled in blankets or heavy clothing.
- Stay out of the heat and humidity by staying indoors during the hottest time of the day (usually mid-morning to mid-afternoon).
- **The use of air conditioners helps ... even for young babies and infants.** If an air conditioner is unavailable, try to stay at the lowest level of the house, as it tends to be cooler. Also, try to keep the house as shaded as possible by closing window, blinds, and curtains. A fan will help as well.
- Do not stay or leave children in parked cars during hot weather.
- Avoid vigorous exercise in the heat (this includes children as well). If you have a young child or a child with a chronic respiratory condition such as asthma, do not allow them to partake in sporting events or exercises during heat waves, especially when there is a heat/humidity advisory in effect.

- Drink plenty of fluids. Water is good. Sports drinks are good too, as they contain added salt. It is important to know that children may not feel thirsty, but will still need to drink regularly. Avoid drinking beverages containing caffeine.
- When in the sun, keep track of how long a child has been outside. Learn to recognize the signs of heat exhaustion right away, so you and your child can get shelter in order to avoid further heat injury. Also, use your common sense and remove your child from the sun and the heat as frequently as you think is necessary. Do not overdo it.
- If your children are swimming in an outdoor pool, a lake, or the ocean, you have to be aware that the high humidity and sunrays are still potential threats. Proper sunscreen protection as well as frequent rests in the shade are still necessary.
- Children are unable to perspire as much as adults are and, therefore, are more prone to heat stress during exercise than adults are. A sensible approach must be used in determining if children can safely partake in sports activities during heat/humidity waves.

### What About Smog During Heat Waves?

Hot, humid air often carries pollutants, pollens, and moulds in higher concentrations than usual. Under these conditions, breathing this air may be harmful to younger children and children with chronic respiratory or cardiac conditions. During smog and heat/humidity alerts, be extra careful by not letting your children outside while the advisory is in effect.

## Mosquito Bite Protection

Here are some ways you can protect your family from mosquito bites. This is particularly important if you live in an area where West Nile Virus occurs.

- Limit time spent outdoors at dawn and dusk, when many mosquitoes are most active.
- Wear light-coloured protective clothing such as long-sleeved shirts, long pants, and a hat when outdoors in areas where mosquitoes are present.
- A long-sleeved shirt with snug collar and cuffs is best. The shirt should be tucked in at the waist. Socks should be tucked over pants, hiking shoes, or boots.
- When going outdoors, use insect repellents that contain DEET or other approved ingredients. Note that insect repellents containing DEET should not be used on infants less than six months of age.
- Make sure that door and window screens fit tightly and have no holes that may allow mosquitoes indoors.
- To avoid insect bites, do not use scented soaps, perfumes, or hair sprays on your children.
- For young babies, mosquito netting is very effective in areas where exposure to mosquitoes is likely. Netting may be used over infant carriers or other areas where young children are placed.

### About DEET

DEET is generally used without any problems. There have been rare reports of side effects, usually, as a result of overuse. The least concentrated product should be used. As with all insect repellents, the product should be applied sparingly and not be applied to the face and hands. Prolonged use should be avoided.

The American Academy of Pediatrics has recommended a concentration of 10 percent DEET or less for children aged between two and twelve. In situations where a high risk of insect bite complications exists, for example West Nile Virus presence in the community, the use of one application per day of DEET may be considered for babies aged older than six months and less than two years of age. Please consult your healthcare provider to discuss the use of DEET or any possible alternatives for your child.

According to the US Centers for Disease Control (CDC), there are no reported adverse events following the use of repellents containing DEET in pregnant or breastfeeding women.

### Precautions When Using DEET

- Read and carefully follow all directions before using the product.
- Young children should not apply DEET to themselves.
- Dress a baby and young child in long sleeves and pants when possible and apply repellent to clothing.
- Apply DEET sparingly only to exposed skin and avoid overapplication. Do not use DEET underneath clothing.
- Do not use DEET on the hands of young children and avoid the eyes and mouth areas.
- Do not apply DEET over cuts, wounds, or irritated skin.
- Wash treated skin with soap and water upon returning indoors. Also, wash treated clothing.
- Avoid using sprays in enclosed areas.
- Do not apply aerosol or pump products directly to the face. Spray your hands and then rub them carefully over the face (avoiding eyes and mouth).
- Do not use DEET near food.
- Keep repellents out of reach of children.
- Do not apply to infants under six months of age.

### Reducing the Mosquito Population Around Your Home

This is an important aspect of mosquito control. Mosquitoes lay eggs in standing water and it takes about four days for the eggs to grow into adults that are ready to fly. Even a small amount of water—like in a saucer under a flowerpot—is enough to act as a breeding ground for mosquitoes.

As a result, it is important to eliminate standing water as much as possible around your property.

- Regularly drain standing water from items like pool covers, saucers under flowerpots, pet bowls, pails, recycle bins, garbage cans, etcetera.
- Drill holes in the bottom of recycling bins.
- Change (or empty) the water in wading pools, birdbaths, pet bowls, and livestock watering tanks twice a week.
- Turn over plastic wading pools and wheelbarrows when not in use.
- Clean and chlorinate your swimming pools. A pool left unattended can produce a large number of mosquitoes.
- Landscape your garden as necessary to eliminate stagnant waters (mosquitoes can breed even in any puddle of water that lasts for more than four days).
- Get rid of unused items that have a tendency to collect water, including old tires.
- Cover rain barrels with screens.
- Clean eavestroughs (roof gutters) regularly to prevent clogs that can trap water.
- If you have an ornamental pond, consider getting fish that will eat mosquito larvae.

## Pedestrian Safety

While more injuries occur at home, the most serious ones are outside the home and result from traffic accidents. Young children are particularly at risk—both as pedestrians and as passengers. I have already talked about protecting your baby in the car, but here are some important precautions that can reduce the risks when taking your baby outside.

When out walking your child, walk defensively. Always stay alert to traffic, establish eye contact with drivers, and obey traffic signals.

Be aware that most pedestrian mishaps occur at dusk and at times when visibility is reduced, so be sure to wear bright or reflective clothing, and consider putting reflectors on the child's stroller.

It is never too early to teach children to be careful when crossing, walking, or playing near streets and traffic. Here are some important habits that should be practised, demonstrated, and taught by parents.

- Teach your children as early as possible that a red light means stop and never to cross on a red light, even when the temptation of no oncoming traffic is there.
- Children less than ten years of age cannot be taught how to cross busy streets safely on their own and, therefore, should always be accompanied.
- Children should be taught never to dart or play between parked cars.
- When walking at night or in the late afternoon (especially at dusk), it is important to wear bright clothing. If you are pushing a stroller, it is a good idea to put glow-in-the-dark or reflective stickers on the stroller.
- As a driver, make sure that the area is clear when you back out of a driveway.
- Children (and parents) should not walk or jog with headphones on. This might result in an accident if you cannot hear what is going on around or behind you.
- Playgrounds around busy traffic areas should always be fenced.

## Petting Zoos

Animals such as cows, goats, sheep, horses, rabbits, pigs, and poultry in petting zoos and on open farms can spread infections to people. Young children are particularly susceptible to these infections.

To protect you and your young children when visiting a petting zoo, wash your hands and your children's hands at these times:

- After touching or feeding an animal;
- After touching an animal's cage;
- After falling or touching the ground;
- Right after leaving the animal areas;
- Before eating or drinking; and
- After cleaning and/or removing boots or shoes.

Also, when you and your children are in the animal areas,

- Don't eat, drink, or chew gum;
- Don't let children lick or suck their fingers or bite their nails;
- Do not let children touch their faces or mouths;
- Do not give babies bottles, pacifiers, or soothers;
- Do not let children kiss or hug the animals.

## Playground Safety

Here are some important facts and tips about playground safety.

- The majority of unintentional injury-related deaths among children occur during evening hours when children are most likely to be out of school and unsupervised. It is important for parents to make sure that their children receive the proper supervision at all times.

- Most playground injuries result from falls. Children can fall off equipment, fall from heights (the top of a slide or a monkey bar), and trip over equipment.
- Drawstrings of hoods and collars of jackets, shirts, and hats can strangle a child if caught on playground equipment. One way to prevent this is to remove the drawstrings from the child's clothing. For similar reasons, scarves should not be worn during play either.
- Make sure that metal slides are cool in order to prevent children's legs from getting burned while sliding down them. Also, check that there are no splinters or nails sticking out on the surface of playground equipment.
- Make sure that there are no rocks, pieces of glass, toys, debris, or other children at the bottom of a playground slide, before allowing your child to use the slide.
- Do not let young children play in areas designated for older children, as the young ones can accidentally get hurt by older children or equipment not meant for them.
- In order to prevent young children from wandering off into heavy traffic areas or streets, playgrounds and play areas should be fenced in.
- After a long winter, playgrounds and other play areas should be inspected for any damage or rust resulting from harsh winter weather wear and tear. Only after inspection and repairs (if necessary) should children be allowed to use these. Also, be sure to refresh your memory with the potential hazards these pose to children and how to prevent them.

## Pool and Outdoor Water Safety

In order to keep swimming fun and safe, it is important to be very careful when children are swimming. Here are some tips and facts about water safety:

- Summer fun includes swimming at the pool or beach. In order to prevent a tragedy, never leave children alone in or near the pool, or beach, even for a second.
- When it comes to pool safety, remember that teaching your child to swim does not mean that your child is safe in the water. So, even if your child has taken swimming lessons, you should still never leave him or her alone in the pool or at the beach.
- At the pool or beach, make sure that anyone watching your children knows CPR (Cardio Pulmonary Resuscitation) and is able to rescue a child if needed. In fact, it is a good idea for parents and other child caregivers to take first aid courses that include CPR training. Also, it is important to keep all rescue equipment by the pool at all times.
- In general, swimming lessons are not recommended for children less than three years of age, as parents may develop a false sense of security by thinking their child can swim. Also young children often swallow pool water, which may be dirty, resulting in a higher risk of getting sick.
- When boating or canoeing, remember that every passenger should always be wearing a life jacket, even if they are good swimmers.
- In addition to pools and the beach, there are other water hazards that could be found near or in your home. They include ditches, postholes, wells, fish ponds, fountains, pails, bath tubs, and toilets. Parents should be aware that these pose a drowning threat

to young, unattended children and they need to watch their children closely if they are playing near any of these areas.

- Children should never swim around anchored boats, in motor boat lanes, or where people are water skiing. Also, they should never swim during electrical storms.
- When buying a life jacket for your child, make sure that it is the right size. The jacket should be snug and not loose, and be worn as per the instructions with all the straps belted properly.
- In order to avoid spinal injuries from diving, swimmers should not dive in shallow areas of lakes, ponds, beaches, streams, and pools where the depth of the water is not known. Also, do not dive into above-ground pools.
- Keep all electrical appliances away from the pool, in order to prevent electric shock during swimming.
- All pools and hot tubs should by surrounded by four-sided fences with self-closing and self-latching gates.
- Do not allow tricycles, bicycles, or other toys on wheels around the pool area.
- Do not think of inflatable toys as life jackets. Floaties are not approved as life jackets and can give children a false sense of security.
- To avoid spread of infection, all pools should be adequately chlorinated. Swimming in pools with inadequate chlorination makes it easier for bacterial infections to spread.
- After pool use, remove all toys from the pool, so children are not tempted to try to reach them. Secure the pool so they cannot get back into it.

## Swimming: Common Questions Parents Have

### At What Age Should a Child Start Learning How to Swim?

According to the Canadian Paediatric Society, swimming programs for infants and toddlers less than four years of age aren't an effective drowning-prevention strategy. It is important to know that children less than four years of age don't have the developmental ability to master water survival skills and swim independently.

### At What Age Can My Child Swim in a Lake or River or Recreational Facilities?

Aside from the drowning dangers, other water facilities pose additional threats to children; these are related to infections. Illnesses can be caused by swallowing, breathing in, or coming in contact with contaminated water from swimming pools, spas, lakes, rivers, and oceans. They include a variety of diseases, such as infections of the gastrointestinal tract, respiratory tract, skin, ear, eye, and existing wounds. Many people don't realize that disease transmission through the use of recreational water can be a serious source of illness. Basically, if a beach or similar swimming area is tested and deemed safe for swimming, children of any age can enjoy it, provided, however, that the following measures are taken:

- Continual one-on-one-supervision.
- Babies and infants should always be in the arms of an adult.
- Ensure that baby's head is kept out of the water so that he or she will not swallow recreational water.
- Do not let your child swim when he or she has diarrhea.
- Wash children thoroughly, especially their bottoms, with soap and water before allowing them to enter the water.

- Wash their hands with soap and water after each bathroom use.
- Wash your hands after each diaper change.
- Change diapers in a bathroom, not by the water.
- Take your child on frequent bathroom breaks and check diapers often.

In all situations, parents and caretakers should use common sense in determining whether the conditions are appropriate for young children to swim.

## Safe Gardening Tips

A garden can be a dangerous place for babies and young children. Prevention is the best approach. Here are some garden safety tips.

- During the annual back yard spring clean-up, make sure that all tools including rakes, scissors, pliers, and cutters are not left lying around, but rather are stored safely out of the reach of children.
- As the snow clears, the backyard pool, although not in use, is still a drowning threat for a young child. Make sure that you take all the necessary safety precautions to avoid a tragic accident.
- When planting bulbs and plants make sure these are out of reach of small children, as some can be poisonous when ingested and others can pose a choking threat if inserted into a young child's mouth.
- To prevent injury from cuts in the yard, parents should make sure that the ground is free of potentially sharp objects such as broken glass. Also teach children to avoid playing in bushes with thorns.
- The outdoor-backyard shed usually contains tools and products that can be very dangerous to children. Always keep the backyard shed or Cabana locked.

## Sun Protection

Protecting a baby from the sun is very important. Indeed, young babies are more prone to the effects of the sun, because they have thinner skin than adults do. As well, babies (when less than six-months old) cannot move themselves out of the sun without a parent's help. Even babies with darker skin are prone to damage from the sun. When I say "damage," I mean a sunburn that is painful and uncomfortable, but I also mean long-term problems. Research now suggests that the more a child is exposed to sun early in life, the higher the chances are that skin cancer develops at an older age. Indeed, the UVA and UVB rays of light are known to cause skin damage which, in the long-term, can become cancerous. So the best way to prevent this long-term potential sun-induced consequence is to protect children and get used to having fun in the sun, but with sun precautions at all times.

It is important to know that the sun's rays can go through clouds, causing damage even on cloudy days. In the shade, the sun's rays can bounce from sand, concrete, or snow, so keep that in mind, as well. In addition, sunglasses with UVA/B protection are also recommended.

What can you do to protect your babies and young children? Well, sunscreens are designed basically to block the sun's rays. The Sun Protection Factor (SPF) is a measure of how much protection the sunscreen offers. For example, an SPF of 30 means that a child can stay out in the sun 30 times longer than without the sunscreen. I usually recommend that a parent or caretaker apply, at the very least, a broad-spectrum sunscreen (one that protect against both UVA and UVB rays) and an SPF of 30. In general, most sunscreens can be used on babies less than six months old, but only on small areas of the body.

Parents should avoid sunscreens that contain PABA (para-aminobenzoic acid) as this may irritate the skin. Sunscreens should be applied thirty minutes before sun exposure, because it takes some time for them to work on the skin. Remember that even sunscreens claiming to be waterproof need to be reapplied every two hours. While putting sunscreen on the face, avoid the eyes. If the sunscreen burns the eyes, try a new type or one that can be applied with a stick applicator. Make sure that all potentially exposed areas are covered including the nose, cheeks, tops of the ears, and the shoulders. Also, never use suntan oil, as it offers no protection and causes the skin to burn more quickly.

### Reiterating Tips on How to Protect Your Child From the Sun

- Babies less than six months of age should be kept out of direct sunlight. Put them in the shade, under a tree, in a stroller, under a canopy, etcetera.
- A baby should be dressed in clothing that covers all of their body (long sleeves, long leg pants, etcetera).
- A cap with a bill is helpful. The bill should be facing forward (not like a catcher in baseball) in order to protect the face.
- Also, tightly woven clothes offer better protection than clothes with a wider weave.
- As children spend more time outdoors than adults do, it is not surprising that most of the exposure to the sun (up to 80 percent) happens before the age of eighteen years.
- When taking your child out to play or for a walk during the spring and summer months, it is important to remember that the sun's rays are the strongest between 10:00 a.m. and 4:00 p.m.
- Parents should be aware that the sun's rays do come through the clouds on cloudy days, so it is important to use sunscreen even when it is cloudy and not sunny.
- Baby oil is not a good suntan lotion. As a matter of fact, baby oil causes the skin to sunburn more quickly and offers no protection at all from the sun's rays.

- If your child gets a sunburn, keep her completely out of the sun until the burn is fully healed.

## Travel Safety

When travelling with babies and small children, it is important to plan ahead. Firstly, make sure that if you are going to a hotel or resort that they are used to having children. When arriving at the hotel, resort, a cottage, or even a friend's or relative's house, make sure that the place is child-safe. Do not take for granted that where you are going will be as child friendly as your home. Make sure your child is not exposed to hotel room hazards including in-room hot tubs or Jacuzzis, hanging curtain cords, wires, open plugs, and the hotel room minibar. Also check that the hot water from the bath and other faucets is not too hot.

Before going on a trip, make sure that you know where the local medical clinics are in case of a medical emergency. It is always a good idea to bring along a first aid kit containing bandages, tweezers, scissors, antibiotic cream, sunscreen, calamine lotion, and acetaminophen.

If your child has a chronic medical problem such as asthma or diabetes, make sure that you discuss your travel plans with your child's healthcare provider and that you know where to go in case he or she needs medical care. It's a good idea to bring along a summary sheet of your child's medical history including a list of medications. Bring along enough medication to last the trip's duration. If travelling by air, pack the medications in a carry-on bag, rather than in the checked luggage.

Remember that it will take longer to drive to your destination with children as compared to driving the same distance alone or just with adults. Make sure that you plan this extra time into your schedule. Bringing along toys, books, games, electronic tablets, laptops, or movies to keep the kids busy during the trip is a good idea. Also, expect to make frequent stops, for bathrooms, stretching, and just getting fresh air.

If your child gets car sick, discuss this with your healthcare provider, as there are some medications that may prevent this. Additionally, there are some other things you can do that can help prevent or reduce car sickness: try to drive at a constant speed, rather than making frequent speed changes; give your child light snacks instead of heavy meals; and keep the windows a bit open to circulate some outside air.

When travelling by plane with young children, ask your airline to make arrangements to accommodate your child in a car seat. Many children have been injured while sitting on a parent's lap in planes during turbulence. Depending on the time of year and whether the flight is fully booked, certain airlines may not charge you for the extra space taken up by the car seat.

### Travel Vaccine and Related Precautions

Vaccinations prevent serious diseases. In general, we have a set of vaccinations that are designed and scheduled based on age, health situation, and our geographic location. However, even if you are up to date with your country's schedule for immunizations, it does not mean that you are protected from diseases found in other parts of the world. This is particularly important when you are travelling outside Canada and the US. For this reason, if you are planning a trip abroad, speak with your healthcare provider or local travel health clinic, regarding the need for vaccinations and other precautions. Each destination has its own particular risks in terms of disease and what vaccines would be required. So during a pre-trip consultation, your health professional will be able to search a database that outlines what the disease risks are for the particular country (or countries) you are travelling to. It is important to prepare in advance as some shots need up to a few months before the complete immunization series can be given. So please plan ahead in order to assure that you are fully protected.

## Some Infections That are Common Abroad

### Hepatitis A

Hepatitis A is a virus that infects the liver, but it is transmitted either through eating contaminated food and drink, or by swallowing contaminated water while swimming. There is no cure for this infection, though it is less dangerous than hepatitis B. There is an effective vaccine for hepatitis A.

### Hepatitis B

Although found worldwide, this infection is very common in Asia. This viral infection of the liver, for which there is no cure, is transmitted through sexual contact and contact with contaminated blood and blood products found on needles and razors. This disease can lead to liver failure, cancer, and even death. There is an effective vaccine for hepatitis B.

### Meningococcal Meningitis

This is a potentially deadly bacterial infection that attacks the covering of the brain and can also cause the body to go into shock. It is spread through respiratory droplets from the nose and throat of an infected person. Although there are antibiotics available for this infection, they are not always fully effective. A meningococcal vaccination is available.

### Typhoid Fever

This is a bacterial infection that can cause severe diarrhea, dehydration, and even death. Typhoid fever is transmitted the same way as hepatitis A, either through eating contaminated food and drink, or by swallowing contaminated water while swimming. There is a vaccine available for this infection.

**Yellow Fever**

This is a potentially deadly viral infection that is transmitted by mosquitoes. There is a vaccine available for this viral infection as well.

**Malaria**

Finally, I want to mention malaria, which is a disease transmitted by a mosquito. This disease kills millions of people worldwide every year, especially in Africa. Although there is no vaccine for malaria, if you are travelling to a region where malaria is endemic (or ever present), you will need to take anti-malarial medications on a preventative basis for the duration of your travels.

Which vaccines and precautions you will need depends on your destinations. So be prepared. Don't forget your travel shots and have a safe and healthy trip!

# Handling and Caring for Baby

A new baby seems so fragile, but this should not scare you as new parents. Get comfortable with holding your baby, and learn the best way to handle him or her. As babies grow and develop and become stronger, handling them becomes easier.

## Baby's Head

Fontanels, also known as soft spots, are openings in the skull where the bones haven't grown together yet. There are two fontanels on your baby's head. The anterior fontanel—on the top of the head—may be as wide as five centimetres (two inches), and is generally closed by the eighteenth month. The posterior fontanel, toward the back of the head, is smaller. It usually closes by about the third month or earlier.

Many parents worry about injuring their baby's soft spot. But below the fontanels, there's a tough membrane that protects the baby's brain. Normal handling of your baby won't injure the fontanels or the brain. Until your baby is strong enough to support him or herself, be sure to always support her head, neck, and back when lifting, carrying, and lowering him or her. By feeling the fontanels, healthcare providers can assess a lot about baby's head growth and certain medical conditions.

## Bathing Baby

It's important to keep your baby clean to lessen the risk of infections and rashes. But a full bath every day isn't necessary. In fact, two or three times a week will be enough until your baby begins to crawl. However, your baby's face, neck, hands, and bottom should be cleaned daily. To make bathing a more pleasant and successful event, choose a time when your baby is calm. Also, avoid bathing a baby who's just been fed—too much handling after a meal may cause her to spit up.

Here are some additional helpful tips for bathing your baby.

- Keep the room that you bathe the baby in warm, so that she isn't chilled. Also, use warm water to bathe her, **never hot**, as hot water may scald baby's sensitive skin. Test the temperature by dipping your elbow in the water.
- Until the umbilical stump has fallen off, avoid tub bathing. Instead, sponge bath your baby or wash him or her with your hands, keeping the stump area as dry as possible.
- When your baby is ready for tub baths, use an infant tub, a plastic dishpan, or a sponge seat made especially for babies. If you're using a sponge seat, be sure to let it dry properly between baths to avoid mildew growth.
- Fill the tub **without** the baby in it, to prevent accidental scalding. The tub should be filled with no more than five centimetres (two inches) of water.
- Never leave your baby alone, even for a moment. So make sure you have everything you need on hand, including soap, shampoo, towel, diaper, and clothing. And be sure to hold baby firmly during the bath.
- When washing, start with the cleanest areas first, and work

toward the dirtiest, so that the washcloth and the water stay clean for as long as possible. After washing each area, be sure to rinse thoroughly.

- Wash your baby's skin with mild soap once or twice a week. Daily use of soap is only necessary on the hands and the diaper area. The rest of your baby's body can just be washed with water on most days, until he or she starts to crawl or is particularly dirty.
- Take special care when washing your baby's face, neck, ears, buttocks, genitals, and folds of skin.
- To clean your baby's ears, wash only the outside of the ear. Never put anything (such as a Q-tip®) into your baby's ear, as this can damage the eardrum and ear canal.
- A baby's hair only needs shampooing with a mild shampoo once or twice a week. Just rinse her hair with water on days between shampooing.
- When cleaning your baby's genitals, use a soft, clean cloth and lukewarm water. For girls, be sure to wash the area from front to back, being careful to gently clean between the folds of skin. Rinse with fresh water.
- No special care is needed to clean a boy's uncircumcised penis. Don't try to pull back the foreskin to clean underneath; this isn't necessary. Simply wash the penis with soap and water.
- Avoid tub bathing a circumcised newborn, until the penis has healed. In the meantime, protect the healing area with a piece of sterile gauze coated with petroleum jelly or an antibacterial ointment. If there are any signs of redness, swelling, bleeding, or pus, be sure to call your healthcare provider.
- After bathing, gently pat dry your baby's skin with a soft towel. Be sure to dry the bottom well, and other areas where there are folds of skin.

## Umbilical Care

Within about one to three weeks after birth, your newborn's umbilical stump will turn black, dry out, and finally fall off. In the meantime, clean the base of the stump two or three times a day with water on a sterile cotton ball or gauze. In order to keep the stump dry, fasten diapers below the navel. Alcohol is no longer recommended. The baby's shirt should also be rolled above the stump, to allow for free circulation of air.

When the cord falls, there may be slight bleeding in the navel area. This isn't any cause for concern and should resolve in two or three days. Be sure to report it to your healthcare provider if you notice any foul smell, reddening, or oozing around the umbilical stump, as well as any bleeding that lasts for more than three days.

## Dressing Baby

For the first week or so after birth, babies can't regulate their own body temperature to adapt to heat or cold as well as adults can, so it's important not to overdress or underdress them. Dress the baby warmly, but not so that he or she is hot. After the first week or two, it is safe to dress your baby more or less as you would yourself.

During cooler weather, baby's feet should be kept warm. Also, dress your baby in several layers of light clothing rather than in a single heavy layer. Several light layers hold in warmth better than a single heavy layer, and they can easily be removed as necessary. When going out, it's a good idea to bring along an extra layer or two, in case your baby needs them.

Hats and caps are also an important part of a baby's wardrobe. During cooler weather, a hat can prevent baby from losing heat through his bare head. In warm weather, a cap protects baby's delicate skin on the head and face from sun exposure. If your baby is underdressed or overdressed, he may fuss or cry. If he is sweaty, he's probably overdressed.

## Baby Carriers

Parents commonly use baby slings and carriers to carry their babies. There are various types available, including soft carriers and harder backpack types. Soft carriers including slings and wraps are for infants less than six months of age. Harder, backpack types that carry baby on the back or the front of a parent are for older children who weigh more than seven kilograms or fifteen pounds and have good neck and head control.

While carriers may be practical, using them incorrectly can lead to injury or suffocation. Serious injuries and deaths can occur if and when:

- The wearer trips and baby falls out of the carrier;
- The product malfunctions or its hardware breaks;
- The baby falls over the side of the sling or out through the leg openings;
- The baby is positioned incorrectly, causing suffocation against the product's fabric, the wearer's body, or their own chest.

Babies born prematurely or with a medical condition are at higher risk of suffocation. Talk to your healthcare provider before using a carrier if this is your situation. Here are some general baby carrier tips to ensure your baby's safety and comfort adapted from Health Canada's website.

- Choose a carrier that is size and weight appropriate for the baby and for the adult who will carry the baby.
- Read the safety recommendations and respect the age, weight, and size limits, and keep the safety guidelines.

- Ensure that the baby carrier hasn't been recalled.
- Make sure your baby is safely placed in the carrier.
- Every time you use the carrier, make sure the stitching is intact and that all ties and straps are in perfect condition.
- When you place baby in the carrier, if it's a shoulder strap carrier, make sure that the knot or buckle is securely tied to avoid the child falling. The guidelines should show examples of safe knots.
- Place baby in a position where he or she can breathe. Make sure baby's chin is not on his or her chest, or that his face is not squeezed against your body. No other objects should be in the carrier that prevent breathing, including a coat, blanket, straps, and clothes.
- While in the carrier, the baby's head and neck should always be straight to allow for proper breathing. Check on baby often to ensure baby is neither in a curled, chin-to-chest position, nor that the face is pressed against you or the carrier material.
- Protect your baby from the cold when you go out in winter. Do not block his breathing with your coat. During warm or hot weather, watch that baby does not get overheated.
- To prevent yourself from falling, make sure there are no objects blocking any stairs.
- Never use soft baby carriers when doing activities that could endanger your baby: for example, cooking, boiling water, biking, driving a car, stepping on a stool, chair, or ladder, jogging, skating, etcetera.
- Never use soft baby carriers in places where you could easily fall, e.g. on icy sidewalks.
- Never sleep or take a nap with your baby in the carrier and never leave a baby alone in the carrier.
- Hold the baby tightly when you bend down to avoid him slipping out, and make sure you don't bump into surrounding objects such as doorframes and posts.

- Make sure that your baby's back is well supported.
- Always carry your baby in an elevated position and very close to your body to distribute weight evenly; this will be less tiring for you.
- Make sure that the openings for the legs are small enough so your baby doesn't slip out through them—but not too tight. You don't want to cut off your baby's blood flow.

These are general guidelines. Which specific type of carrier you use depends on your individual situation, needs, and preferences. Regardless of which type you choose, always follow the manufacturer's specific recommendations and guidelines.

# Getting Used to Baby's Routines

The arrival of a new baby certainly changes a family's routine. Parents very quickly realize that their newborn's patterns may not fit with their usual family routines prior to their baby's arrival. The good news is that most parents get to know their newborn very quickly and get used to his new routines and needs, many of which change over time. This is yet another good reason for parents to get close and bond with new baby as soon and as much as possible. Though these early routines can be challenging for new parents to adapt to, it helps to realize how much your newborn needs you, and that things will soon become a lot more normal. I hope this section can help you understand some of the new routines and characteristics a new baby presents. As I said, you will get used to them quickly, especially if you learn about, understand, and expect them ahead of time.

## Vital Signs

Vital signs refer to a person's heart rate, respiratory rate, blood pressure, and temperature. Vital signs of a baby are usually checked at birth and during routine physical examination or when a baby is being evaluated for a medical problem. Abnormal vital signs usually signal that there is something wrong. Some parents are unaware that normal vital sign values or ranges in babies and young children vary with age and differ from those of adults.

The pulse or heart rate of a newborn is quite rapid as compared to an adult. At birth, the heart rate can normally be as high as 140 to 150 beats per minute; at two years of age, still as high as 120 beats per minute; and by about eight years of age, a child's heart rate reaches the adult rate of between 70 and 80 beats per minute.

A newborn's respiratory rate—the number of breaths they take per minute—is also high. It is between 35 and 50 breaths per minute, as compared to the adult rate of about 18 to 20 breaths per minute. Breathing may be irregular in young babies; in other words, the baby may take a few breaths, then pause for a few seconds, then continue again. This is normal, as they develop and mature their breathing. Just like with heart rate, the respiratory rate decreases as a child grows.

A baby's blood pressure is much lower than in adults. According to the *Nelson Textbook of Pediatrics*, the normal blood pressure range of a newborn is between 65/45 mmHg and 85/55 mmHg. At one year of age, the normal range of blood pressure is between 90/55 mmHg and 105/70 mmHg. As a baby grows, the blood pressure increases gradually and reaches adult levels by about twelve years of age.

# Crying Patterns

As a pediatrician, I am very aware that babies often cry, and at times to the point where parents become worried and upset. The good news is that crying during the first few months of life is common and part of a baby's normal development. Indeed, some babies seem to cry a lot and nothing helps. During this phase of a baby's life, they can cry for hours and still be healthy and normal. Parents often worry that there is something wrong. However, even after a checkup from the doctor that shows the baby is healthy, baby continues to cry for hours, night after night. In extreme situations, a crying baby can be a source of tremendous frustration for parents and caregivers. Sadly, at times, a parent or other caregiver may shake their baby out of desperation or even anger. Please remember: **never shake a baby** as this can cause serious brain damage or even death.

## The PURPLE Period of Crying

If parents understand that bouts of crying, especially during the first few months of life, are normal, they will be less frustrated and be more comfortable with their infant. In fact, all babies go through what is called the PURPLE period of crying. This concept was created by a mentor and colleague of mine, developmental pediatrician, Dr. Ron Barr. Dr. Barr's approach is to explain this phase to parents of newborns to encourage them so that they know it is normal and that it will end. This knowledge can reduce parental frustration, anger, and any tendency to shake a baby.

The acronym "PURPLE" is used to describe specific characteristics of an infant's crying during this phase. The word "period" is important because it signals that this phase is temporary and will end eventually. Each letter of the word "PURPLE" stands for something that describes this period of crying, something that is essentially seen in all babies to some degree:

- **P: Peak of Crying**—Baby may cry more each week. They tend to cry more at two months and then less at three to five months.
- **U: Unexpected**—Crying can come and go, and you do not know why.
- **R: Resists Soothing**—Baby may not stop crying, no matter what you try.
- **P: Painlike Face**—A crying baby may look like they are in pain, even when they are not.
- **L: Long-Lasting**—Crying can last as much as five hours a day, or more.
- **E: Evening**—Baby may cry more during the late afternoon or evening. I refer to this as a crying shift.

Essentially, all babies go through this period when their crying peaks at about two months of age. Yet every baby differs by the intensity of the crying during this period. Some babies cry more intensely than others do during this time period, while others cry, but less intensely at the same age. In fact, unsoothable or intense crying represents about 5 percent to 15 percent of all crying and fussing that infants do. Excessive crying can be seen in all babies, no matter if they are breastfed or formula fed.

If you or someone you know has a newborn baby that is crying a lot, it is important to understand that in most cases, this is normal. Knowing more about your baby and the period of PURPLE crying will lessen your frustration and worries, and allow you to fully enjoy your new family addition! For more information, please visit www.purplecrying.info.

In addition to the above, crying may be a way babies express their needs such as being hungry, being tired, or needing a diaper change. Different types or sounds of crying mean different things. Parents will soon discover this and understand what to do. As babies grow older, and become better able to express themselves through other forms of communication, they will cry less often, and for shorter periods of time.

## Coping With Crying

Although crying is not usually a cause for alarm, it can be stressful for parents, caregivers, and the baby. Keeping baby's environment peaceful and calm, particularly around feeding time, and in the late afternoon and evening may help prevent or minimize crying episodes. When your baby does cry, be sure to respond. Don't just let baby cry. Babies who are left to cry may begin to feel abandoned and insecure, and are often harder to calm. As I said before they need TLC for their brain to develop normally, so don't worry—babies can't be spoiled at this age! Based on what science tells us today, babies who are given a lot of attention in the first few months tend to be happier, healthier, and better adjusted in the long run.

### Strategies to Calm a Crying Baby

- Wrap your baby snugly in a blanket. Many babies find this soothing. But remember, never put your baby to sleep with a blanket wrap. This is sometimes called swaddling (see section below).
- Gently pick your baby up and rock her in your arms.
- Singing softly or gently massaging their tummy or back seems to soothe many babies.
- Babies love gentle rhythmic motion. Go for a walk outdoors together using a stroller, baby carrier, or just your arms—it may calm your baby while providing some much needed stress relief for you too! Or if you prefer, strap your baby into the car seat for a ride in the car; this may help calm or lull him or her to sleep.

### Swaddling Your Baby

Swaddling is thought to mimic the enclosed feeling a baby experiences in the womb during pregnancy and has become quite popular. According to the American Academy of Pediatrics, when done correctly, swaddling can help calm babies and promote their sleep. However, there are a few important facts and guidelines that parents need to know about and follow to ensure safe swaddling. Done incorrectly, swaddling can result in overheating and hip problems. So it is important to ensure that baby's hips can move and that the blanket is not too tight. You should be able to fit at least two to three fingers between the chest and the blanket. Also, swaddled babies can roll over onto their stomachs and suffocate. This is why babies who are swaddled should be placed only on their back and watched closely so that they do not roll over accidentally. Swaddling should stop by two months of age

### When Nothing Soothes Your Baby

Sometimes, nothing will soothe a crying infant, and the episode will need to simply run its course before crying will subside. Though it may be difficult in these circumstances, it's important that parents try to remain calm, both for their own sake and for the sake of their baby. Babies can sense their parents' anxiety and nervousness, and this may upset them further, leading to more intense crying.

If your baby's crying jags are leaving you feeling stressed or burned out, leave the baby in the hands of a competent babysitter, and take time out for a movie, a dinner out, or just a few hours of quiet relaxation! You'll come back revitalized, better able to cope, and feeling like you've missed your baby.

## When Is Crying a Sign of Something Wrong?

Sometimes, crying indicates a serious problem. If your baby's cries are unusual (they don't follow the usual pattern) and are accompanied by fever, vomiting, diarrhea, or other signs of being unwell, you should seek medical attention immediately. The same is true of a baby who normally does not cry much, but suddenly has an episode of sustained, high-pitched crying, or screaming. These signs could indicate a serious medical problem needing immediate attention.

## Feeding Patterns

Generally, babies fed mother's milk will want to feed about twelve times a day, while babies fed with a milk formula usually demand eight feedings per day. In the coming months, baby will eat increasingly larger meals, faster, and a little less often. Although each baby is different, the number of feedings per twenty-four hours varies with age. Here is a table adapted from the *Nelson Textbook of Pediatrics*:

### Average Number of Feedings per 24 Hours by Age

| Age | Number of feedings |
|---|---|
| Birth to 1 week | 6 to 10 |
| 1 week to 1 month | 6 to 8 |
| 1 to 3 months | 5 to 6 |
| 3 to 7 months | 4 to 5 |
| 4 to 9 months | 3 to 4 |
| 8 to 18 months | 3 |

I have a quick rule of thumb that I use as a very general reference. I call it the Rule of Four. By four months, a baby usually needs four meals per twenty-four hour day. Remember that this varies with each baby, but it can give parents a general idea of what is usually seen by this age.

After each feeding, your baby should be burped in order to expel any air that might have been swallowed along with the breast milk or formula. If the swallowed air isn't expelled, it can cause discomfort and your baby may spit up. To burp your infant, hold her upright against your chest and shoulder, and gently rub or pat her on the back. You can also burp her while holding her in a sitting position on your lap. It's a good idea to drape a towel or cloth diaper over your shoulder or on your lap, because your baby may spit up a little milk along with the air. More detailed information on feeding your baby will be discussed in the nutrition section of this book.

## Sleep Patterns

On average, most newborn infants sleep about sixteen and a half hours per day, but some may sleep as little as nine hours, and others as much as twenty-two hours per day. Infants tend to sleep for short periods of about two hours, and then wake for about thirty minutes before falling back to sleep. Others may nap for shorter periods while some may soon sleep for stretches of five or six hours.

The parents of a newborn are likely to have their own sleep patterns upset. This is normal and only temporary. But it is also helpful to know that babies who are awake to feed every three hours during the day and evening are likely to be less wakeful during the night.

In the coming months your baby will nap less often, but for increasingly longer periods. And by about the sixth month, your child will likely sleep through the whole night and remain awake much of the day.

| **Age** | **Total hours of sleep** | **Day time hours of sleep (naps)** |
|---|---|---|
| 1 week | 16.5 | 8 |
| 1 month | 15.5 | 6 |
| 3 months | 15 | 5 |
| 6 months | 14.25 | 3 to 4 |
| 9 months | 14 | 3 |
| 12 months | 13.75 | 2 to 3 |
| 18 months | 13.5 | 2 |
| 2 years | 13 | 1 to 2 |
| 3 years | 12 | 1 |
| 4 years | 11.5 | - |
| 5 years | 11 | - |

## Ensuring Good Sleep Patterns/Habits: The Earlier the Better

Sleep problems are among the most common complaints that parents have about their young children. Needless to say, they can cause a lot of stress in the family. Kids end up tired and parents become exhausted from being up all night with the baby.

Typically, children with sleeping problems do not fall asleep easily and also wake up in the middle of the night. Whether a sleep pattern or habit is abnormal depends on the age of the child. Sleep patterns in babies take time to develop into normal sleep cycles of being asleep for the full night and awake during the day. In fact, most babies do not develop normal sleep patterns, until about four to six months of age.

Most sleep problems develop when parents react too quickly to a child who is fussy at night, not realising that baby, if left alone for a few minutes, may indeed fall asleep by herself. When a parent reacts immediately to a first cry, baby gets used to being comforted. Not surprisingly, the baby soon learns to expect attention immediately.

*NOTE: In my section on Coping With Crying, when I am discussing prolonged crying episodes that tend to occur in the evening or late afternoon, I recommend that parents respond to a crying baby. When a baby is put to bed for night-time sleep, we can take a slightly different approach so that baby can learn to go to sleep on her own. If she initially cries or fusses upon being put to bed for the night, I think it is fine to let her alone for a few minutes as long as the crying is decreasing and she eventually falls asleep. If, however, after a few minutes, and I mean only just a few minutes, the crying continues or intensifies, parents need to respond. I do not believe in the sleep training method of letting them cry it out for as long as necessary to fall asleep.*

Here are some simple tips recommended by the American Academy of Pediatrics to prevent sleep problems:

- Keep baby as calm as possible by avoiding too much stimulation during the night so she can fall back asleep easily.
- Try not to let baby sleep as long during the day.
- As soon as baby is tired, put her to bed immediately. In this way the baby will learn to relax herself to sleep.
- Rocking or holding a baby until she falls asleep creates a habit. Soon the baby will need to be held and comforted back to sleep every time she wakes in the middle of the night.
- Avoid putting baby to bed with a pacifier. A pacifier helps to soothe the baby, but the baby should not get used to sleeping with it.
- Do not put the baby to sleep in your bed. Aside from the risk this may pose to your baby, this can also create poor sleep habits and, consequently, sleep problems.

One very important thing that parents and caregivers can do is make sure that they are well rested. When you are fresh and relaxed, you can cope better with your baby's situation. Of course, that's not always easy. One helpful tip is, if possible, to take turns with your partner to get up with the baby. Alternating with your spouse/partner will help ensure that at least one of you is reasonably well rested. A good night's sleep will give you a bright new perspective in the morning. Perhaps the most crucial thing to remember in creating good sleep habits in a child is consistency. All persons providing care for a baby should be in sync with the approach and be very consistent when trying to deal with, or help prevent, a sleep pattern problem.

# Bowel and Urination Patterns

During the first six weeks, newborns will have at least one bowel movement per day and as many as fifteen. Newborns urinate up to ten times per day.

## What Is Normal?

Normal bowel and urinary function varies considerably from baby to baby. Regularity and frequency of bowel movements varies not only between babies, it can even change in the same baby from day to day.

Stool frequency in breastfed babies can vary from as many as fifteen per day to just one bowel movement every few days, after a few weeks. The passing of only one stool every few days does not necessarily indicate constipation. Neither does grunting, pushing, or turning red in the face while passing a stool. This is normal behaviour, as long as stools are soft, do not contain blood, and do not appear to be causing pain.

The colour, consistency, and odour of bowel movements also vary with age and diet. In the first few days of life, your baby's stool will likely be greenish-black and sticky. This is called meconium. Over the next few weeks, your infant's stool will likely be semi-liquid and green-brown. The semi-liquid consistency of stools at this age is normal, and shouldn't be confused with diarrhea, in which stools are abnormally frequent and very watery.

After about the third week, the stools of breastfed babies tend to be orangey-yellow, fairly loose and watery, and have a sweet-sour smell. However, stool colour can vary, from yellow to orange, to green, to brown—all of which are usually considered normal.

Stools of formula-fed babies at this age tend be pale brown and somewhat more solid. The odour of stools of formula-fed babies is generally stronger than with breastfed babies, and varies with different types of formula.

As babies grow older, they have fewer bowel movements, and their stools become more formed or pasty. This becomes more pronounced when solids are introduced into the diet. I often get a lot of questions about stool colour and I tell parents that there is no one normal colour. In fact, it can range, as I explained above. Any streaks of blood or mucus in a baby's stool should be evaluated. The only two colours—aside from blood red —that I worry about are if the stool is completely white or completely black. These two stool colours may indicate a serious condition and parents should seek medical attention immediately.

Newborns generally urinate up to ten times per day. Urine typically ranges in colour from clear to pale yellow, and has little or no odour. As the baby grows older, she will urinate less frequently, but in larger amounts. An odour of ammonia may become more apparent in the urine. The longer the urine is left in the child's diaper, the more intense the odour becomes. Blood in a baby's urine may indicate infection and should be evaluated.

Consult your healthcare provider if there are any sudden variations in the pattern of your baby's bowel or urinary habits.

# NUTRITION

One of the most common preoccupations of new parents is feeding and nutrition. This is a very important concern, as newborn babies have unique nutritional requirements in order to support the rapid growth and development of their brains and bodies. What babies eat and drink during the first year of life can have a major impact on their present and future health. However, with time, you will get used to recognizing when baby is hungry, how much is enough, and, by knowing in advance when a certain food or a solid should be started, you can be comfortable in changing your baby's nutrition. After all, during the first few years, aside from growing and developing at a very rapid pace, a baby's capacity to eat, their nutritional needs, and amounts needs change quickly as well. As we are coming to understand the value of good nutrition, it is important to establish good eating habits from a young age. It is never too early to teach children the value of avoiding high fat foods and the importance of fibre, calcium, iron, and other minerals in the diet. Understanding the value of and adapting a well-balanced diet at an early age has lifelong benefits.

Parents often wonder when an infant is able to taste. It is interesting to know that the taste sensation is present from birth and that babies prefer sweetness over saltiness or plain water.

Another common question is: How many calories per day does a baby need to grow normally? On average, babies need between 80-120 calories per kilogram of body weight, per 24-hour day (35-55 calories per pound) during the first year. If you want to calculate roughly how many calories your child needs daily, a good rule of thumb for children up to five years of age is to begin with a base of 1,000 calories and add 100 calories for each year of your child's age. For example: A one-year-old would need approximately 1000 + 100 calories for one year, or 1100 calories per day. A two-year-old would need 1000 + 200 calories for two years, or 1200 calories per day. With this simple equation, you can calculate the approximate number of calories your child needs in order to maintain normal growth.

## Breastfeeding: Best for Baby

The World Health Organization's (WHO's) position is that breast milk is sufficient nutrition for the first six months of life. Some of the many advantages of breastfeeding include protection against infection, helping protect against Sudden Infant Death Syndrome (SIDS), and lowering the risk of childhood obesity. There are numerous nutritional benefits also, as breast milk contains all the necessary nutrients to support and ensure normal growth and development. From the social standpoint, breastfeeding promotes mother-infant bonding. As I explained in the beginning of this book, breastfeeding provides almost all the forms of stimulation that a baby needs to grow and sculpt her brain as normally as possible. This may explain why studies have suggested that breastfed babies have higher IQs than babies not breastfed.

Breastfeeding is very inexpensive, practical, and quite portable. It is not necessary to purchase bottles, infant formula, or other accessories. From the ecological point of view, breastfeeding is very environmentally friendly. As well, according to the American Academy of Pediatrics, there are numerous benefits of breastfeeding to the mother. These include quicker and easier recovery from childbirth and reduced rates of breast and ovarian cancer later in life. Some studies have also shown that breastfeeding mothers have a reduced risk of developing type 2 diabetes, rheumatoid arthritis, and cardiovascular disease, including high blood pressure and high cholesterol.

### Breast Milk: Baby's Ideal Food

Breastfeeding is by far the oldest and most natural way to feed your baby. Breast milk is made up of a complex composition of proteins, fatty acids, sugars such as lactose, amino acids, iron, and many other nutrients tailored to meet your baby's specific and changing needs. In particular, the type of fat in breast milk is naturally ideal for brain and nerve growth and development. These nutrients are delivered in forms that are easily absorbed by your baby's delicate digestive system. In addition, breast milk is made up of easily digestible and easily absorbable protein, fat, and iron. As a result, digestive upsets are uncommon in breastfed infants.

Another major benefit of breast milk is protection against infections—of the intestines, ears, and elsewhere—because it contains antibodies. Antibodies are substances created by the immune system to fight off germs such as bacteria and viruses. Antibodies created in the mother's system are passed through breast milk into the baby's system, offering temporary protection against common infections.

Breast milk satisfies both hunger and thirst. Extra water is usually not needed. Babies fed at the breast control the quantity of milk they drink, drawing as much milk as they desire at a time. As a result, overfeeding and underfeeding are unlikely to occur. Sucking at the breast also promotes good mouth and jaw development. Also, breast milk is always sterile or free of germs.

It is recommended that babies be exclusively breastfed for at least six months. Beyond this, breastfeeding can continue if both mother and baby desire. When taken in combination with solid foods, breast milk is also an excellent source of nutrition for infants older than six months. If your baby is exclusively breastfed, depending on where you live, a Vitamin D supplement may be recommended.

### Colostrum, Foremilk, and Hindmilk

While the content of breast milk changes over the course of baby's development, there are essentially three types of breast milk: colostrum, foremilk, and hindmilk.

*Colostrum* is the yellowish breast fluid that the mother's breast produces in the first few days after baby's birth and before normal lactation begins. Colostrum is especially rich in nutrients and antibodies, and is the perfect food for a newborn baby.

*Foremilk* is the milk that is first drawn during a feeding. It is generally thin and lower in fat content, satisfying the baby's thirst and liquid needs.

*Hindmilk* is the milk that follows foremilk during a feeding. It is richer in fat content and is high in calories. Make sure to let your baby drain one breast before moving on to the other, to ensure that he or she receives the benefits of both foremilk and hindmilk.

## Practical Tips for the Breastfeeding Mother

Generally, babies fed mother's milk will initially want to feed up to about twelve times a day. In the coming months, your baby will eat increasingly larger meals, faster, and a little less often. It's not uncommon for a breastfeeding mother to experience discomfort at first, until her breasts become used to nursing. **Please do not give up**; it is worth the effort!

Here are some practical tips that can help make breastfeeding easier:

- If you have inverted nipples, you may need to pull them out or wear special breast shields to help them protrude, so your baby's mouth can properly latch on to your breast.
- To prevent breast engorgement, feed your baby often and as soon as she is hungry. Also, express or let out some milk if your breasts are overfilled or hard, before you feed baby.
- If your nipples are cracked or sore, expose them to air as much as possible, especially after nursing. This will speed healing and help to toughen them. Also, for the first while, wearing breast shields will allow air to surround the nipple, and will protect them from clothing and other irritations. This won't be necessary once your nipples are accustomed to nursing.

- Don't use commercial lotions or lubricants on your nipples, as they may cause or increase irritation. Also, breastfeeding mothers should wash their nipples with water only. Soap is unnecessary.
- Many breastfeeding mothers wonder if their baby is getting enough milk. It may seem at first that your baby is hardly nursing at all. But rest assured that it's normal for your baby not to drink a lot during the first few days after birth, as she doesn't yet need much milk. By the third and fourth day, your breasts will begin to produce more milk and your baby will also start to drink more.
- Once your baby has begun to feed more, be sure to give baby both breasts and empty at least one at each feeding. It takes at least ten minutes to empty a breast. Your baby will need to feed at least eight to twelve times in twenty-four hours, and shouldn't go more than three hours during the day and five hours at night without a feeding. If your baby doesn't demand a feeding during this time, you may need to encourage him.
- At two to three weeks, there is often a growth spurt, and your baby may seem to be incredibly hungry. Feed your baby as often as she demands. In the coming months, your baby will eat increasingly fewer but larger meals.
- Avoid pacifiers and bottle feeding during the first four to six weeks, so baby can get used to and establish a good breastfeeding routine.

## Taking Care of Mom's Needs

It's important for the breastfeeding mother to maintain a healthy diet and lifestyle, both for her own good and to ensure that baby is getting the healthiest breast milk possible. The following are general guidelines for breastfeeding mothers:

- Follow Canada's Food Guide, the US Food Guide Pyramid, and equivalent guidelines depending on where you live.
- Make sure to drink six to eight glasses of liquid daily to replenish the fluids lost during breastfeeding and be sure to get lots of rest.
- Eat an extra five hundred calories a day of nutritious food, to support your supply of breast milk. The extra calories will not cause you to gain weight. In fact, you may find that you lose weight in spite of your increased food intake.
- It is likely that you will need to take iron supplements to replenish the iron transferred to breast milk. Consult your healthcare provider for advice.
- Avoid foods that seem to be irritating your baby. Limit caffeine and alcohol intake, as these are passed on in breast milk.
- Consult your healthcare provider about taking any prescription or over-the-counter medications, as these may pass through your breast milk to your baby. It's best to avoid taking medications altogether, unless absolutely necessary.
- Don't smoke, and avoid second-hand smoke. Smoking can cause vomiting, diarrhea, and restlessness in your breastfed baby. It may also cause reduced milk production.

## Is Baby Drinking Enough?

The best way to be sure that babies are getting enough milk is by following their weight gain. On average, during the first three months of life, babies gain about one kilogram or two pounds per month. This equals about thirty grams (one ounce) per day. Between the third and sixth months, babies gain about half the amount they gained during the first three months or about fifteen grams (half an ounce) a day. In general, babies weigh double their birth weight by about four months. If your baby is gaining weight and growing normally, you can rest assured that he or she is getting enough milk. Other ways you can tell if baby is getting enough is by the number of wet diapers and the colour of baby's urine. Breastfed newborns who are receiving enough milk generally urinate up to six to eight times a day, and will have anywhere from one to twelve bowel movements each day. Urine should be clear to pale yellow, and have little or no odour.

Although most babies adapt to the breast very well and drink enough, it is important to recognize the symptoms of dehydration that indicate that baby is not getting enough milk. These include:

- Urinating less than normal;
- Darker urine than usual;
- A sunken anterior fontanel;
- Weight loss or poor weight gain;
- Very little or no saliva;
- Unusual drowsiness or lethargy.

**If your baby has any of these symptoms, get medical help immediately. Dehydration can be very dangerous in infants and young children.**

## Expressing and Storing Breast Milk

You may wish to express and store your breast milk occasionally. Stored breast milk can be used by a babysitter when you're unavailable, or by a partner who wishes to share in feeding your baby. A variety of breast pumps is available on the market, which can express milk easily and quickly.

Bottles and containers used to store breast milk should be sterilized or washed in very hot soapy water to avoid contaminating the milk with germs. Be sure to label and date containers storing breast milk, and discard any milk stored for too long. Here are some tips on how to store and prepare your expressed milk from the American Academy of Pediatrics:

- Always wash your hands before expressing or handling your milk.
- Be sure to use only clean containers to store expressed milk. Try to use screw cap bottles, hard plastic cups with tight caps, or special heavy nursery bags that can be used to feed your baby. Do not use ordinary plastic storage bags or formula bottle bags for storing expressed milk.
- Use sealed and chilled milk within twenty-four hours if possible.
- Freeze milk if you will not be using it within twenty-four hours. Expressed breast milk can be stored at room temperature for up to ten hours and in the refrigerator for up to eight days at 0° F to 3.9° C (or 32° F to 39° F). Frozen expressed breast milk can be kept in the freezer compartment located inside a refrigerator for up to two weeks, and for six to twelve months in a self-contained freezer (connected on top of or on the side of the refrigerator) at -18° C (or 0° F ) or in a deep stand-alone freezer at -20° C (or 4° F).
- Store it at the back of the freezer and never in the door section. Make sure to label the milk with the date that you freeze it. Use the oldest milk first.
- Freeze two to four ounces of milk at a time, because that is the average amount of a single feeding. However, you may want some smaller amounts for some occasions.
- Do not add fresh milk to already frozen milk in a storage container.
- You may thaw milk in the refrigerator or you can thaw it more quickly by swirling it in a bowl of warm water.
- Do not use microwave ovens to heat bottles, because they do not heat them evenly. Uneven heating can easily scald your baby or damage the milk. Bottles can also explode if left in the microwave too long. Excessive heat can destroy important proteins and vitamins in the milk.

- Milk thawed in the refrigerator must be used within twenty-four hours.
- Do not refreeze your milk and do not save milk from a partly used bottle for use at another feeding.

## Modern Day Issues

A modern day issue that has arisen with the evolution of both parents working is breastfeeding at the workplace and/or providing time for working mothers to express and collect their milk at work. Actually, this should be considered a right of all working mothers. The advantages extend beyond those mentioned above. By allowing mothers to breastfeed or to express their milk at work, job satisfaction and hence productivity will increase to everyone's benefit, including the employers.

Breastfeeding publicly has been a source of controversy. There was a recent incident in a large Canadian city where a mother was asked to leave a shopping mall by security because she was breastfeeding. I think that anyone who perceives breastfeeding in public places as obscene or indecent is very wrong.

Mothers are urged to protect their right to breastfeed their child in public places and should support places, centres, and malls that allow them to do so. Not only should breastfeeding be allowed in public places, I think that they should facilitate breastfeeding on their premises. The fewer barriers to breastfeeding, the longer it will continue.

## Weaning Baby

Weaning off the breast is a natural process in a baby's development. It usually begins when an infant starts to eat solid foods, but again this varies from baby to baby. Base the decision of when and how to wean your baby on the needs of the mother and baby. My recommendation is that beyond six months of age, babies should continue to breastfeed for as long as possible and practical.

There are several ways a mother can wean baby off the breast: abruptly, temporarily, or partially. Natural weaning occurs when baby gradually becomes less interested in breastfeeding, usually between one and three years of age. If you abruptly or suddenly wean baby (cold turkey), you should pump your breasts to extract the remaining milk to prevent engorgement and plugged ducts. The following general suggestions can help make weaning a positive experience for mother and baby:

- Warm the nipple of the bottle.
- Use expressed breast milk in a bottle.
- Place baby in a different position than when breastfeeding.
- Offer the bottle while baby is happy.
- Do not wait until the baby is hungry.

Remember: if baby becomes frustrated or upset, take a break for a few days before trying the bottle again.

## Formula Feeding

Although it is strongly recommended that babies are breastfed exclusively for the first six months of life, some mothers may choose an alternative to breast milk for a variety of reasons or may start to wean baby before the first six months of age.

The American Academy of Paediatrics recommends that during the first twelve months of life, the **only** acceptable alternative to breast milk is commercial iron-fortified infant formula. Babies should be fed either breast milk or formula, or a combination of both, for the first year. This recommendation may vary in other countries, for example in Canada the current guidelines state babies should be fed either breast milk or formula, or a combination of both, for the first nine to twelve months of life. I recommend you ask your local healthcare provider if you live outside the US and Canada. The bottom line is that cow's milk is not suitable for most or all of the first year of life.

### Why Not Whole Cow's Milk?

Regular cow's milk is not suitable at all for your baby during most or all of the first year. There are many reasons for this. The protein content in regular milk is too high for a baby's intestine to digest and for the kidneys to eliminate. In addition, regular milk can irritate a baby's intestine and is not a very good source of iron. In particular, cow's milk does not contain enough iron to support baby's growing needs. Iron is an essential mineral the body uses to produce blood and other cells. Iron-deficiency anemia can occur if your baby doesn't have enough iron in his system. Anemia during the first year can delay long-term mental and physical development. So it's important that your child is fed either breast milk or iron-fortified formula, not cow's milk, during his first twelve months.

Today, commercial infant formulas are designed to imitate the content and performance of human milk, as much as is scientifically possible. However, it hasn't been possible to create a formula perfectly identical to breast milk. Breast milk is a complex combination of living cells, hormones, enzymes, antibodies, and compounds with unique structures that can't be replicated in a formula.

If you're considering using formula to feed your baby, consult your healthcare provider about the type of formula that is best suited for your baby's particular needs. Formulas should be iron-fortified and contain the recommended levels of other vitamins and minerals.

Parents often ask about or even use 2 percent or skimmed cow's milk. Two percent and skim milk are not suitable during the first two years. If you do not breastfeed your child during the most or all of the first year, feed your baby infant formula. In addition, soy, rice, or any other plant-based drink—even when fortified—are not nutritionally complete and so are unsuitable for babies as a breast milk substitute.

## Definition and Description of the Formulas

So that you'll better understand what milk formulas are, let's discuss the basic components of milk. Generally speaking, breast milk, whole cow's milk, and milk formulas contain milk protein, fat, water, and carbohydrate (sugar), in addition to vitamins and minerals. One way these types of milk differ is the composition or makeup of their protein. Breast milk contains human milk protein, whereas whole cow's milk and regular formulas contain cow's milk protein. The cow's milk protein in formula is modified so it's easier for a child twelve months or less to digest. Another important component of milk is the carbohydrate or sugar. The main sugar in breast milk, whole cow's milk, and regular formulas is the same: lactose.

## Practical Issues When Bottle Feeding

Commercial formulas come in a variety of forms. Ready-made types come in disposable, sterile bottles, or in cans for pouring into bottles at home. Concentrated and powdered formulas are also popular, and tend to be less expensive. These need to be diluted and poured into bottles before serving. Be sure to read instructions for these types of formula carefully. It's very important that directions for mixing be followed exactly. Incorrectly mixed formula can result in malnutrition if the powder is too diluted. Formula that is made too concentrated can also be dangerous as it is too difficult for a baby's system to metabolize.

For your baby's first three months, water used in formula should be sterilized by boiling it. Many people aren't aware that bottled water is not sterile. If you use bottled water to mix your baby's formula, boil it first as you would with tap water. No matter which type of formula you use, always check packaging for the expiration date. Discard any formula that is past due. Storage instructions should be read and followed carefully. Do not reuse formula that is left over in the bottle after a feeding—it can easily become contaminated with bacteria.

Bottles and containers used to prepare formula should be sterilized or washed in very hot soapy water to avoid contaminating the milk with germs. Never warm formula on the stove or in the microwave. Excessive heat can destroy important nutrients in the milk, and can burn your baby's mouth. Microwaves are particularly dangerous as they heat unevenly, often giving a false impression of the actual temperature of the milk. Formula can be served at room temperature, or warmed slightly by immersing the bottle in lukewarm water, then shaking it to distribute the heat evenly.

A word of caution: Never leave your baby with a propped bottle. This could cause your baby to choke. Also, never put baby to bed with the bottle as this can also cause choking, lead to dental cavities, and possibly ear infections. Until your baby has developed the coordination to hold the bottle themself, parents need to hold both the baby and the bottle during feeding times.

## How Much Formula Does My Baby Need?

During the first few weeks, formula-fed babies need to drink between 160 ml and 200 ml per kilogram of their weight (between 2.5 ounces and 3 ounces of formula per pound of their weight) daily.

The average amount a baby drinks per feeding increases with age. Here are the average amounts per feed by age of baby adapted from the *Nelson Textbook of Pediatrics*:

### Amounts of Milk per Feed

| Age | Ounces | Millilitres |
|---|---|---|
| 1 to 2 weeks | 2 to 3 | 60 to 90 |
| 2 weeks to 2 months | 4 to 5 | 120 to 150 |
| 2 to 3 months | 5 to 6 | 150 to 180 |
| 3 to 4 months | 6 to 7 | 180 to 210 |
| 5 to 12 months | 7 to 8 | 210 to 240 |

In addition, initially, baby will need to drink quite frequently. As she gets older, she'll feed less often, but will drink more at each feeding. During the first week, your baby may have six to ten feeds per twenty-four hour period, six to eight per day by one month, five to six per day by three months, four to five per day between three and seven months, and three per day after eight months of age.

## Soy-Based Formulas

For a variety of reasons, mostly related to allergies to cow's milk protein, some babies may be put on soy-based infant formulas. The protein in these formulas comes from soybeans instead of cow's milk. These formulas are also lactose-free. Just like cow's-milk-based formulas, soy-based formulas contain all the necessary nutrients (including iron fortification, adequate fat, and calcium) and calories required for normal growth and development. Children grow and develop normally on soy-based formulas.

Soy-based formula should not be confused with the kind of soy beverages or drinks found in the dairy section of grocery stores. Soy-based formulas are a good substitute for milk-based formulas and cow's milk generally during the first two years—but soy beverages are not.

Note that soy-based formula feeding does not prevent a baby from developing allergies.

# Food Safety Precautions

Before I talk about solid foods, I want to take some time to review some basic food safety habits that will go a long way in preventing your new baby and your family from getting foodborne illness (food poisoning). As you start to prepare baby's foods, even purées, it is important to understand how to prevent foodborne illness, which can be dangerous for all members of your family, but especially to babies and young children.

Foodborne illness is caused by eating or drinking contaminated food or beverage. Most foodborne illnesses are caused by microscopic, disease-causing organisms such as bacteria, viruses, and parasites. However, bacteria are the leading cause of foodborne illnesses.

## Bacterial Food Poisoning

Some types of bacteria grow in food and in your digestive system once you eat the contaminated food. *Salmonella* is a common example of this type of bacteria. It is most often found in poultry, pork, water, and unpasteurized milk.

Other types of bacteria produce toxins. *E. Coli (Escherichia coli)* is an example of bacteria that can produce toxins. Some toxins can lead to severe and fatal illness. The *E. Coli* bacteria can be found in undercooked meat (especially in ground beef), as well as in untreated water or within a defective water treatment system.

### How Can Foodborne Illnesses Be Prevented?

- Wash your hands very well
  - after handling raw meat, poultry, fish, and fresh produce,
  - before eating,
  - after using the washroom, and
  - after changing a diaper .

- Encourage frequent hand washing among all family members.
- Cook and reheat foods very well, to 74° C (165° F) or higher.
- Refrigerate foods promptly at 4° C (40° F) or lower.
- Freeze foods properly at minus 18° C (0° F) or lower.
- Keep your kitchen clean by washing counters, cutting boards, knives, and other equipment after each meal.
- Sanitize counters, cutting boards, knives, and other equipment with a mild bleach solution.

## Picnic and BBQ Safety

Before you know it, you will be taking your young child out for BBQs and picnics. It is also important to take the necessary precautions to ensure that family picnic and BBQ meals are safe too. Here are some important safety and cooking tips:

### BBQ Safety

- When barbecuing, make sure that your young child is far enough away from the broiler in order to prevent a burn injury.
- Keep all barbecue accessories including charcoal, lighter fluid, and propane gas tanks well out of the reach of children at all times.
- Ensure that your BBQ is well maintained and cleaned regularly.

### BBQ Cooking Tips

- Thaw and marinate meats in the refrigerator. The safest method is to place frozen meat, poultry, or fish in a dish in the refrigerator for thawing. Make sure the sides of the dish are high enough to catch all the juices as the food thaws. Place thawing meat on the lowest shelf in your refrigerator to prevent its juices from contaminating other foods. Thawing in the refrigerator takes a lot of time, ten hours per kilo or 4½ hours per pound of meat, poultry, or fish.

- Remember that even if the food has been frozen, this does not mean bacteria have been killed. The meat still needs to be cooked properly. Remember, if you are cooking frozen hamburger patties, you will need more cooking time to reach the proper temperature.
- Use clean utensils and work surfaces to prepare foods.
- Don't serve cooked meats on the same plate that was used for the raw meat.
- Use utensils to handle raw meat and another clean set of utensils to serve cooked meats.
- Cook all meats thoroughly, especially chicken and hamburger. These meats must be well done; they cannot be eaten rare or medium. Use a thermometer to ensure that these foods are cooked properly.
- Eat as soon as everything is cooked.

### Picnic Safety

- Use safe foods as much as possible, such as fruits, vegetables, bread, crackers, and canned goods, rather than foods that require refrigeration.
- Use ice or ice packs in an insulated cooler to keep foods chilled when transporting them.
- Place drinks and snacks in different containers. Since people reach for drinks more often, the main meal will stay cooler longer by being kept separate.
- Cover or wrap food to protect it from insects.
- Discard leftovers that have been left unrefrigerated for two hours or more.

## Introducing Solid Foods

New parents often ask when to start feeding their babies solid foods. In general, babies younger than four months of age should not be given any solids. Here is why babies are not ready for solids before four months:

- Their intestines are not ready to digest solids;
- A baby's mouth and swallowing coordination and reflexes are not fully developed;
- Saliva production is not adequate to help swallowing;
- A baby's control of his head and body is still weak, making swallowing solids difficult.
- Breastfeeding babies do not need to start solids until six months of age. One of the most important reasons to start solids is that beyond six months, breast milk does not contain enough iron for a baby to grow.
- Most experts agree that solid food can begin to be introduced into baby's diet around four to six months. Each baby is unique, so it is important to discuss the specific timing of starting solids with your healthcare provider who knows you and your child very well. At the appropriate age, formula-fed babies should be on cereals regardless of the daily amount of formula taken.

### Practical Points

Iron-fortified single grain cereals should be introduced first as they are easily digested and are an important source of iron. Commercial baby cereals are also heavily enriched with important B vitamins, and are specially designed for a young baby's delicate digestive system. They are also convenient, as they're precooked; you need only add water, breast milk, or formula, depending on the brand. If you choose to use commercial cereals, be sure to read and follow mixing instructions carefully. Plain rice cereal is usually well tolerated and so is often recommended for the first cereal.

Solids should be introduced slowly, and one at a time, so that baby can get used to each new taste and sensation. Also, introducing food slowly allows you to watch for any reactions. Start with one teaspoon of cereal in the morning and one at supper. Gradually increase the quantity if your baby responds well to the food. Try a variety of fortified cereals, one at a time for a week each, so that baby can get used to each new taste and sensation. Watch for any adverse reactions.

If your baby tends to be constipated, avoid rice cereal. Instead, use oatmeal cereal, which has a slight laxative effect. Cereal should be mixed thin at first, until your baby is comfortable with this new food, then mixed thicker as directed. Serve it to your baby with a feeding spoon or other small spoon, which fits easily into his or her mouth. Never put cereal into your baby's bottle.

### When Baby Pushes the Food Back Out

When baby pushes the food back out, it does not mean that she does not like the food. It's a natural reaction for babies to push out their tongues when something is put into their mouths. This is known as the extrusion reflex and is present until about three or four months of age. Baby has not yet developed the control to push it to the back of the mouth, so it can be swallowed—something that will come with practice. It may take a week or more to develop this coordination. In the meantime, it may help to feed baby only a small spoonful of cereal at a time.

### Introducing Other Foods

Once your baby has become accustomed to cereals, try introducing bland puréed vegetables, such as peas and carrots. After a couple of weeks, you can try a variety of fruit purées, although it's recommended that you introduce fruit only after your baby has become used to vegetables. Your baby may not be interested in vegetables after becoming accustomed to the sweeter taste of fruits. Fruit purées can be followed in later weeks by puréed poultry, meat, tofu, or cottage cheese. Be sure to consult your healthcare provider for details about which foods are appropriate for your baby.

Commercially strained baby foods are convenient and popular, but by around six or seven months, your baby can probably handle table foods that have been properly prepared. All home-prepared foods should be puréed until your baby develops adequate mouth coordination to mash or chew more textured or lumpy foods, at around eight months of age. The transition to lumpier or more textured (but still soft) foods should be gradual, and pieces of food should never be large enough to lodge in your baby's throat and cause choking.

Here are some more tips for successful feeding:

- Try to introduce new foods under favourable and pleasant circumstances—not in a hurried or tense fashion, or when your baby is overtired.
- Introduce new solids one at a time for a period of five to seven days each, to observe your child for any adverse reactions.
- If your baby seems to dislike a particular taste or type of food, don't force it. Wait, then try a little bit again the next day. If baby still isn't interested, move on to other foods. After a month or so has passed, try introducing it again, perhaps prepared differently this time. If the food is still rejected, leave it alone. Forcing baby can turn eating into a battle of wills, which can in turn lead to eating disorders. A better approach is to offer other healthy food alternatives.

### Finger Foods

As your baby gets older and starts to have some teeth (between seven and eleven months), small pieces of soft food can be placed on the high chair tray during a family meal. By seeing finger foods within reach, babies can learn to pick up the pieces and feed themselves and will get used to eating with the rest of the family. Note that this should only be done under constant supervision and once your baby has teeth and you ensure that the pieces offered are small enough so he will not choke. Almost any food that is healthy and nutritious and has a soft texture makes for a good finger food, if it's cut small enough. It may take some time for your baby to get the hang of it, but don't worry, he will love it!

## Common Nutrition Related Issues

### Giving Juice to Baby

I do not recommend giving juice to your baby until she is older than six months of age. If you do start giving her juice, limit the amount she drinks to about five to six ounces daily. On average, infants drink about five ounces of juice per day, most commonly apple or grape. At this amount, there is usually no problem. However, excessive amounts of juice can decrease a child's appetite and in some rare cases cause abdominal discomfort and related symptoms. Also, it is important to opt for natural juices instead of fruit drinks, which are just sugar-sweetened, fruit-flavoured beverages.

### Giving Baby Water

Babies really do not need water during their first six months of life, because breast milk and/or baby formula contains all the water they need. If you do choose to give baby some water, for babies less than three months old, boil tap water first to sterilize it. Also, bottled water is not sterile and for this age group would need to be boiled first. If children over six months of age want to drink water, you can give them a few sips, but make sure it does not fill them up to the point where they will not be hungry.

### Homemade Foods for Baby

Many parents prefer making their baby's food at home as they can choose and control what they're feeding their baby. It is also cheaper than commercially made preparations and it gets infants used to eating the same food the rest of the family enjoys. When preparing foods, make sure you wash and rinse your hands and equipment, and clean fruits and vegetables well. In general, any fruit, vegetable, or meat (without skin) can be puréed or mashed (for older toddlers). There are many recipes and ideas online. Once you have prepared the food, ensure that you store it in airtight containers that are labelled with the date and the name of the type of food.

### Should Any Foods Be Avoided To Prevent Allergies?

In the past, we recommended waiting until babies were older than one year before feeding them certain highly allergenic foods, like eggs, fish, or berries, especially if there is a family history of allergies. However, new research has found that introducing these foods to children under the age of one does not increase their chances to become allergic to them. The current recommendations state that these allergenic foods can be given to babies before their first birthday. In cases where there is significant family history of food allergies, particularly to peanuts or shellfish, some pediatricians would still recommend not introducing these foods during the first year and perhaps would even suggest waiting longer. If this is your case, please speak to your healthcare provider.

## Vegetarian Diets for Baby

Vegetarianism is becoming increasingly popular. There are four main categories of vegetarians:

- Ovolactovegetarians consume eggs, milk, and plant foods.
- Ovovegetarians consume eggs and plant foods.
- Lactovegetarians consume only milk (or other dairy products) and plant foods, but do not eat eggs.
- Vegans eat plant foods only.

As a child's growth and activity vary with age, so do their dietary needs. Therefore, the possible effects of a vegetarian diet depend on the child's stage of development. During early childhood and beyond, vegetarian diets can meet a child's needs if properly balanced and/or by taking the appropriate supplements.

Needless to say, if you are a vegetarian and you want your child to be one, you need to recognize there are some potential deficiencies that should be prevented. For instance, it is important to make sure that your child is receiving enough calories to grow. Some vegetables are bulky and may fill an older children, so they will be less hungry and not eat enough calories overall to support growth.

Assuring that there is enough protein in the diet is extremely important as well. Protein is the only source of essential amino acids, which are vital for normal growth. To ensure enough protein intake, parents should learn which foods are high in protein content and use these in all meals. High-protein foods include beans and other legumes.

Calcium deficiency also needs to be prevented. Good sources of calcium include soy products such as tofu, and green vegetables such as mustard greens and broccoli. Vitamin D deficiency is possible especially in ovovegetarian and vegan diets and may need to be supplemented.

Although zinc is plentiful in animal muscle, it may be inadequate in vegetarian diets. Aside from zinc supplementation, zinc can be found in beans, whole grains, and some green vegetables.

Iron deficiency can be prevented by eating foods high in iron such as beans, whole grains, green vegetables, and dried fruits such as prunes and peaches. It is a good idea to go over a vegetarian child's diet with your healthcare provider or nutritionist to prevent any potential nutritional deficiency.

I have gone through the possible nutritional deficiencies of vegetarian diets in children, but there is no doubt that there are very substantial, lifelong benefits to a properly balanced and supplemented vegetarian diet. Adult vegetarians tend to be less fat, have lower cholesterol, have lower blood pressure, less constipation, and less osteoporosis than adults who eat meat-containing diets. A vegetarian way of life is not a bad thing to get a child used to, especially knowing the associated definite long-term health benefits. Adults often have trouble changing their lifelong eating habits. It is easier if we learn to eat more healthfully as infants and young children.

## Vitamin Use

Basically in today's North American society, the following recommendations for vitamin supplementation are generally applied to full-term, healthy babies and toddlers eating well-balanced diets.

- Exclusively breastfed babies generally need to take a daily vitamin D supplement (400 IU) depending on the area they live in. If your baby is partially breastfed and partially formula-fed, the same recommendation applies.
- Formula-fed babies do not need any vitamin supplementation.
- Fluoride drops may be recommended depending on where you live and the age of your baby. Your healthcare provider or your

municipality's water authority will be able to provide you with the fluoride content in your local water. When given regularly at a young age, fluoride has been shown to significantly reduce dental cavities. Again, whether a baby needs fluoride or not, and how much, if any, depends on the fluoride content in your local drinking water.

If your baby was born prematurely, or has any chronic medical condition, vitamins and perhaps other nutritional supplements may be necessary. Your healthcare provider will be able to give you specific details based on your baby's individual situation.

### Switching From Bottle to Cup

Most experts agree that the age to switch from bottle to cup should be between twelve and eighteen months. It is sometimes difficult to do, so you may have to eliminate the bottle gradually. To make things easier, eliminate the mid-day bottle first, then the evening and morning ones. Eliminate the night or bedtime bottle last, as it is usually the one most difficult to stop.

# Growth and Development

## Babies Are Different From Adults

Before discussing specifics about baby's growth and development patterns, I want to discuss the field of pediatrics and how taking care of children differs from taking care of adults. In general, there are many types of primary healthcare providers who take care of babies and children, including pediatricians, family doctors, nurses, and nurse practitioners. Technically, the field of pediatrics covers all aspects of taking care of children's medical needs. However, it's more than just following and treating sick children. Pediatric practice is equally devoted to following and ensuring the normal growth and development (both physical and mental) of children from birth through adolescence (eighteen years of age). Healthcare providers caring for children deal with a constantly changing patient population. When a child is born, he or she grows from a seven-pound baby to a one-year-old who's walking and talking. During the routine checkups, healthcare providers follow these changes making sure they occur normally. In addition, providers also help in disease and injury prevention by providing immunization (vaccination) and educating parents on health-related issues and safety/environmental preventative awareness that will protect children from injury and ensure normal growth and development.

One of the challenges in caring for babies and very young children is that they don't speak and, therefore, cannot communicate verbally. Healthcare providers must obtain the necessary details from the parents or caregivers. Additionally, any treatment, although intended for the child, needs to be fully explained to the parents who themselves administer it. I refer to this as medicine by proxy: treating children through an intermediary. On the other hand, when dealing with older children and adults, the treatment and communication occurs directly between the healthcare provider and the patient.

The following summarizes the key roles of healthcare providers working with a pediatric population:

- Ensure normal growth and development, including physical and psycho-social-emotional development.
- Help in the prevention of illness and injury.
- Diagnose and treat (follow, if necessary) children with illnesses or other conditions.
- Provide the necessary support, information, and resources so that parents can understand as much as possible about their children's growth, development, safety, and overall health and wellness.

An important way to help ensure your baby is growing normally is to schedule regular checkups. Because growth and development are important signs of a child's health, and because changes occur so rapidly during the first eighteen months, checkups need to be organized on a frequent, regular basis during this important period of your child's life. At these checkups, your healthcare provider measures and tracks your baby's growth and development. Your baby's height, weight, and head growth are recorded on a growth curve and monitored carefully. A growth curve is a chart that illustrates the average rate and amount of growth in children within the same age range. As children get older, checkups to assess growth and development are generally only necessary every six months, or once a year.

## Growth Rates During the First Two Years of Life

During infancy and childhood, there are many important physical and developmental changes that take place, especially in the first year and a half of life. During this time, baby's brain and body grow at a tremendous rate. At birth, the average baby weighs about 3.25 kilograms or 7 pounds and measures about 50 centimetres or 20 inches. Note that during the first week of life, it is normal for newborns to lose up to 10 percent of their birth weight. After this temporary weight loss, by seven to eight days of age, babies starts to gain weight regularly. By four months of age, babies usually weigh twice as much as their birth weight. By one year of age, the average baby will likely weigh about three times as much as at birth—about 10 kilograms (22 pounds) and measure about 75 centimetres (30 inches) in height.

During the second year, growth slows down and baby may only gain about 2.5 kilograms or between 5 and 6 pounds, and grow in length by about 12 centimetres or 5 inches. The average eighteen-month-old weighs between 10.5 and 11 kilograms or 23 and 24 pounds, and measures about 85 centimetres or between 33 to 34 inches tall.

I want to stress these are averages and there are some babies who will grow at faster rates while others grow at slower rates. This is why we use growth curves that, very importantly, track the rate and pattern of growth.

### Growth Curves

When a child is assessed for growth, three important measurements are taken: height, weight, and head circumference. These measurements are then placed or plotted on a growth curve or chart that illustrates the average rate and amount of growth in children within different age groups. In other words, growth curves allow your healthcare provider to record and follow baby's specific pattern of growth. Whether a baby is growing normally or not depends on the rate of growth over time as compared with the average or normal rates for that age. Because boys grow at different rates from girls, separate growth curves are used for each gender. In order to be able to properly assess a child's growth, the curve has to be maintained and looked at over several measurements and time. In this way, the growth curve really charts out a child's growth pattern and rate until adulthood. Consequently, the growth curve is a vital part of any child's medical record.

Growth curves can also provide very good clues as to whether certain problems or symptoms are serious. For example, a common complaint is that a child is not eating enough or is a picky eater. How serious or worrisome the problem is depends in large part on the growth pattern. If the growth rate is normal, then despite the picky eating habits, the child is getting enough calories to grow. Similarly, when assessing babies and young children for other problems such as frequent infections or colds, an important part of the assessment is looking at the growth curve. Again, if the growth rate is normal, chances are that there really is nothing seriously wrong. The growth curve is a child's, parent's, and the healthcare provider's best friend. However, a growth curve can only be kept up to date when parents bring their children in for regular checkups.

It is important to understand that each child is unique. Parents should not compare one child to another. This is not the purpose of growth charts; their role is to help make sure that a child is growing at a normal rate.

The growth charts previously used up until a few years ago reflected an American population. The WHO charts better reflect the global profile now by representing a broader global population range

Note that certain conditions or situations are associated with different growth rates and patterns: babies born prematurely and children with chronic medical conditions display different growth rates. As a result, specific growth charts are currently available for children with specific situations and conditions, such as premature birth and Down's syndrome.

## Head Growth

One of the important parts of a pediatric checkup, especially during the first eighteen months of life is measuring the size of a baby's head. A baby's head is large in comparison to the rest of its body. The neck muscles are too weak to support the weight of her head—so it's important that parents and caregivers support her head when picking her up or holding her. By the third or fourth month, she will be strong enough to hold her head up without support.

Head growth occurs at its most rapid rate during the first year of life, then grows at a slower pace.

Importantly, head circumference growth is an indirect measure of brain growth and development. The skull of a baby is made up of several bones that are not fully joined to allow for this growth. The head circumference is taken by placing a measuring tape around the child's head above the forehead. Both the actual size of the head and, more importantly, the rate at which it grows are important components of the routine baby checkup.

### What Can Go Wrong?

If the head is too large or growing too quickly or, on the other hand, if the head is too small or growing too slowly, these are signs of possible problems.

Before worrying about the actual size of the head, we need to focus on the growth rate. Looking at just one value in time is difficult as we need to assess the growth pattern. This is best done by plotting the head circumference on a chart, much in the same way as the height and weight are recorded and followed at each pediatric checkup. A normal growth rate pattern is a key sign that things are normal.

If the head circumference is smaller than the lower limit of normal range, but the rate of growth is normal, then we think of "familial microcrania," a term that refers to a tendency for members of the baby's family to have smaller heads, where growth and development occur perfectly normally otherwise. In this case, a measurement of the parents' head sizes often shows that one of them has a small head.

The same is true for a larger than normal head in a baby who otherwise follows a normal pattern or growth rate: This is known as familial macrocrania or a large head that runs in the family. Again, one of the parents will likely have a larger than normal head.

One other important aspect of evaluating the head growth is ensuring that the fontanels (soft spots) do not close prematurely. Normally the posterior fontanel closes on its own by three to four months, and the anterior fontanel closes by the eighteenth month. If they close earlier, it may signal a possible problem, where the skull bones connect and fuse earlier than they are supposed to. This serious situation can prevent the head and brain from growing normally. Although not all cases of premature closure of the fontanels are problematic, **they all need to be assessed** with an x-ray and in some situations by a neurosurgeon. If there is an associated skull bone fusion abnormality, it will likely require a surgical correction. Fortunately, in my practice most babies with premature closure of the fontanels are well otherwise, have normal skull x-rays and their heads grow normally. It is important to have your baby's head circumference measured regularly. It is really the rate of growth of the head that we want to focus on, rather than the actual size itself. In this way, we can screen for both the slowing down or acceleration of head growth, both of which are conditions that need prompt (in some cases, urgent) investigation and attention.

# Developmental Milestones

## The First Eighteen Months of Development

Being there for baby's first smile, first steps, and first words are wonderful experiences, and keeping a record of these firsts can be fun and informative. Studies have shown that in healthy full-term children, "developmental milestones" are generally always achieved within certain age ranges. An important part of the general pediatric checkup is to make sure that your baby is reaching these developmental milestones.

At birth, a baby's arms and legs are curled close to his body, like they were in his mom's womb. As the baby's muscles develop, his limbs will uncurl, and he will have better control over movements. By their second or third month, babies discover their hands and become increasingly fascinated by them. And as their hands start to unclench, they will be able to grasp objects. At about the same time, babies are able to push themselves up on their arms. By the third or fourth month, they learn to roll over. With this ability, babies can move surprisingly far and fast, so they should be constantly supervised to keep them safe.

By about the seventh month of age, babies may be able to sit unsupported and pull themselves up to a standing position using a chair or other surface. Around this time, the baby learns to crawl. However, it is also not unusual for a baby to progress from sitting straight into walking (skipping the crawling phase), somewhere around their first birthday. It also not unusual for babies to take their first steps as late as eighteen months.

## Developmental Milestones by Age

The following is a more detailed list of milestones or abilities children have at different stages of their development during the first eighteen months of life. It's important to remember that these are only general guidelines, and that babies are unique individuals who can develop at quite different rates and still be healthy and normal.

## From Birth to Two Months

During the first two months, babies' senses develop as they slowly begin to awaken to the outside world. Loud noises will cause them to startle, cry, or become very quiet. Their hands will unfurl and may grasp your finger. Babies' eyes will focus on close objects, such as a toy or your face. To the parents' delight, babies will sometimes smile when talked to or touched. Babies will also begin to coo and gurgle, and by the end of the second month, may be able to lift their head and chest off the floor for brief periods, using their forearms for support.

**Developmental Milestones For a Baby From Birth to Two Months**

- Reacts to loud noises.
- Grasps your finger.
- Eyes focus on close objects.
- Smiles.
- Coos and gurgles.
- Lifts head and chest briefly, using forearms as support.

## Babies Aged Two to Three Months

Between two and three months of age, babies will learn to lift their heads more steadily and for longer periods. They will become more active, moving their limbs and exploring their hands and feet. They are able to reach for objects close by and even grasp them. Babies will also start to put things in their mouth to explore them, so be sure that objects within their reach do not pose a choking hazard. When placed on their tummies, babies at this age can prop themselves on their forearms and raise their upper body higher. They are interested in faces and the sound of voices and become increasingly aware of other members of the family.

**Developmental Milestones for a Baby Aged Two to Three Months**

- Lifts head more steadily and for longer.
- Becomes more active.
- Reaches for and grasps nearby objects.
- Puts objects in mouth.
- Props himself on his forearms, raises upper body.
- Is interested in voices and faces.

## Babies Aged Four to Five Months

By age four to five months old, babies have increasing muscle control. They are able to reach easily for things, bring their hands together, and pass objects from one hand to the other. While on their stomachs, they can sometimes roll over onto their back and vice versa. They have fun by playing with their own feet and hands. Babies at this age can also sit up, but still need back support. In these months, your baby will also become more alert and may fuss if bored or wanting attention. She reacts when you smile at her or call her name, and she is able to follow you with her eyes. Babies at this age look for the source of sounds and also learn to laugh.

**Developmental Milestones for a Baby Aged Four to Five Months**

- Reaches easily.
- Passes objects from one hand to the other.

- Rolls over in one direction.
- Plays with feet and hands.
- Can sit up with support.
- Demands attention.
- Reacts when you call his/her name.
- Looks for the source of sounds.
- Laughs.

## Babies Aged Six to Seven Months

By six and seven months, your baby will probably be able to sit up without support. He will also be able to get up on all fours and rock back and forth. This is practice for crawling in the coming months. Babies can now also roll over both ways easily. By this age, babies are able to pick things up with their fingers, so be careful to keep dangerous objects out of their reach. Babies will be able to feed themselves, look for something that has dropped, imitate sounds, and babble.

**Developmental Milestones for a Baby Aged Six to Seven Months**

- Sits up unsupported.
- Gets up on all fours.
- Rolls over easily both ways.
- Rakes items up with fingers.
- Feeds him or herself.
- Looks for something that has dropped.
- Imitates sounds and babbles.

## Babies Aged Eight to Nine Months

During their eighth or ninth month, babies can easily move into a sitting position from their stomach and become more mobile, crawling or scooting around. They may begin to pull themselves up into a standing position while holding onto furniture, and from there, they may start to cruise around furniture. It's very important to remember to babyproof your house before your baby starts crawling or cruising, to ensure that the environment is safe and free of potential hazards.

In addition to becoming more mobile, baby's eye and hand coordination also improves at about this time. They are now able to pick up small objects with their thumb and forefinger in a pincer grasp. Your baby is also starting to understand cause and effect. For example, if she pushes a button on a toy, music plays. A baby may also begin to experience separation anxiety at about this time, and become upset when she is separated from you, even briefly.

**Developmental Milestones for a Baby Aged Eight to Nine Months**

- Moves into sitting position from stomach.
- Becomes more mobile; crawling or scooting.
- Pulls up into standing position while holding onto something.
- Begins to cruise furniture.
- Uses pincer grasp to pick up objects.
- Understands cause and effect.
- May experience separation anxiety.

## Babies Aged Ten to Eleven Months

By ten to eleven months, your baby is becoming more and more independent, crawls, and wants to explore everywhere. He may stand on his own for brief periods of time. He may also begin to take steps while holding onto mom's or dad's hand, and enjoys playing peek-a-boo, and filling up and emptying containers.

**Developmental Milestones for a Baby Aged Ten to Eleven Months**

- More and more independent.
- Stands unaided for brief periods.
- Takes steps holding mom's or dad's hand.
- Plays peek-a-boo.
- Enjoys filling up and emptying containers.

## Babies Aged Twelve Months

By twelve months of age, babies begin to climb and can now reach objects that were previously out of reach. So you'll need to watch your baby carefully and keep dangerous objects safely away. Babies will also take their first step by themselves at about this time. By one year of age, babies can say, "Mama" and "Dada," and use simple gestures such as shaking their head or waving bye-bye. Baby can also understand "No," and possibly a few other basic words.

**Developmental Milestones for a Baby Aged Twelve Months**

- Climbs.
- Starts to take independent steps.
- Says "Mama" and "Dada."
- Uses simple gestures.
- Understands "No" and some other basic words.

## Babies Aged Fifteen Months

By fifteen months of age, baby will probably be walking unaided and seem to become very busy at this time, and less interested in eating and sleeping. Dexterity (movement and coordination of her hands) has improved, and she can now turn door handles, unscrew container tops, and feed herself with a spoon. At this age, your baby enjoys splashing in water, playing in the sand, and has learned a few more words.

**Developmental Milestones for a Baby Aged Fifteen Months**

- Walks unaided.
- Improved dexterity.
- Feeds herself with a spoon.
- Enjoys splashing water and playing in the sand.
- Says a few more words.

## Babies Aged Eighteen Months

By eighteen months, your baby will be moving around with greater ease and control, and begin to climb stairs. She will also be able to scribble with a crayon, turn the pages of a book, and point to a body part. Vocabulary will increase to several words, and she will pretend to talk on the telephone.

**Developmental Milestones for Babies Aged Eighteen Months**

- Climbs stairs.
- Scribbles with a crayon.
- Turns the pages of a book.
- Points to a body part.
- Says several words.
- Pretends to talk on the telephone.

# Supporting Baby's Physical and Emotional Development

## TLC, Affection, Attention, and Stimulation

Parents play a critical role in supporting and encouraging baby's healthy growth and development. One of the most important ways parents can do this is to give plenty of love and attention. As I described in the beginning of this book, science now very clearly tells us that for a baby to develop to their full potential, physically, mentally, and emotionally, the most important ingredients of their care during the first few years of life are attention, love, and stimulation. Healthy parental and caregiver relationships with your baby will help his brain to wire positively and develop the necessary connections resulting in healthy and well lives. I mean healthy life in the holistic way. This encompasses a child's physical wellness along with their emotional and mental wellness. This holistically healthy and well upbringing will collectively allow for the ability to control their emotions, to relate positively with others, and to learn and prosper to their full potential over the course of their entire lives.

So hold, hug, touch, and encourage your baby as often as you can. By being affectionate with and responsive to your baby, you'll help build baby's sense of security as she or he learns to explore the world and at the same time lay the foundation for a prosperous and healthy life.

## Learning Through Play

Another vital part of your baby's development is learning through play. When you play together, baby is learning, developing, having fun, and bonding with you, all at the same time! Be sure to set aside time to play with your baby often.

During this segment, I describe how you can stimulate your baby's development through playful interaction and the use of age-appropriate, baby-safe toys. Note that toys do not need to be expensive or complicated to be fun and stimulating. So be creative by also playing with common household items such as boxes, pots and pans, plastic utensils, and bowls. Just be sure that all items baby plays with do not present any potential choking hazard or have sharp edges. Remember that babies love to interact with you, but they love to explore things by themselves as well. So leave them some time and opportunity to play and explore and discover on their own too.

In the beginning of the book, I discussed the benefits of reading to babies. I highly recommend that you find as much time as you can to read to your baby in addition to the activities listed here. Invite others to read to baby, too, like grandmother, big brother, or sister. Anytime we read to babies is just another investment in their vocabulary, future learning ability, and success!

## Birth to Four Months

From birth to four months, you can encourage your baby's social development by talking often to him or her, and responding to his or her gurgling and cooing. This will help your baby begin to learn the basics of conversation. Your baby will also enjoy your singing and humming. To help stimulate physical development, gently move your baby's limbs. Place babies often on their tummy, and position a toy or baby-safe mirror in front of them to encourage them to lift their head and look up. Offer rattles or other toys your baby can grasp and play with. Because babies are putting things in their mouths at this age, it's very important to be sure that all toys and objects within her reach are baby-safe, and do not have small pieces that can come off easily. Toys should be marked as appropriate for this age, and pose no choking hazard.

### Toys Appropriate for Babies From Birth to Four Months Old

- Rattles;
- Rings with plastic objects attached to them;
- Images or books with high-contrast patterns;
- A colourful mobile above baby's crib;
- Colourful objects of different textures, sizes, and shapes;
- Musical toys;
- Non-breakable baby mirror.

## Four to Eight Months

You can encourage baby's development at this stage by giving him plenty of attention and stimulation, as well as some quiet time. Talk to your baby often as you dress, feed, and play with him. Imitate the sounds he makes. Read him simple books with large images. Hang or place brightly coloured objects within baby's reach, which baby can look at, touch, and turn. Let your baby feel many different textures. Help him learn to sit by propping him, under close supervision, in the corner of a chair or a couch where he can't fall over. Your baby will enjoy building block towers with you and knocking them over. Play pat-a-cake and other hand games, and bounce a favourite toy just beyond baby's reach to encourage him to try and get at the toy.

### Toys Appropriate for Babies Aged Four to Eight Months

- Soft balls;
- Toys that have finger holds;
- Baby books with board, cloth, or vinyl pages;
- Musical toys;
- Activity boards that include objects that can be handled, turned, and moved, and that make sounds;

- Large cloth, wood, or plastic blocks;
- Toy telephones;
- Spoons and measuring cups;
- Bath toys.

## Eight to Twelve Months

Between eight and twelve months, your baby is becoming increasingly mobile and curious. Let her move around to explore the environment, but be sure to babyproof any areas that she can now reach. Continue to encourage developing crawling and cruising skills by placing toys in front of baby, just beyond her reach. Help her walk holding onto your hands. Roll a ball to her, and ask her to roll it back to you. Be sure to give plenty of praise and applause. She will also enjoy looking at picture books. Encourage language skill development by pointing out and naming the pictures.

### Toys Appropriate for Babies Aged Eight to Twelve Months

- Picture books;
- Plastic pails, cups, and other unbreakable containers;
- Colourful, washable toys such as balls, plastic blocks, stacking rings, and stuffed animals;
- Large dolls and puppets;
- Squeezable toys;
- Cars, trucks, and other similar toys with wheels, as long as they are made of flexible plastic and have no sharp or removable parts;
- Toy instruments and other musical toys.

## Twelve to Eighteen Months

Between twelve and eighteen months, you can encourage your baby's growing language skills by playing word games. Ask, "Where is your nose? Your mouth? Where is your foot?" And be sure to give him plenty of praise when he's correct. Also, continue reading to your baby regularly. Babies enjoy lift-the-flap and touch-and-feel books at this age.

To encourage fine motor skills, give your baby paper and crayons to scribble. You can put him in a highchair to do this, to prevent scribbling on walls and furniture. He will also enjoy toys that can be stacked or taken apart and put back together.

During this time, your baby's balance and coordination improve as he masters walking and other gross motor skills. You can support his development by demonstrating how push-and-pull toys work, and dancing together to music. Help him learn to climb stairs safely by letting him practise with your supervision. Show him how to get down stairs on his tummy. Of course, never leave him unattended, and also use gates at the top and bottom of stairways.

Your baby will also love wagons, cars, and other riding toys. Babies at this age also love to play hide-and-seek.

### Toys Appropriate for Babies Aged Twelve to Eighteen Months

- Lift-the-flap and touch-and-feel books;
- Large non-toxic crayons;
- Beginner jigsaw puzzles;
- Shape sorter games;
- Push and pull toys;
- Digging toys such as shovels and buckets;
- Outdoor toys such as swings, slides, and ride-on toys (meeting all current safety standards for this age).

# Vision, Hearing, and Tooth Development

## Vision

During the first eight weeks, a baby's vision is very nearsighted and their eyes may often seem to be crossed. By the second month your baby's vision will be improved enough to recognize familiar faces, like Mom's and Dad's, at which time you'll probably also see your child's first smiles. By the fourth month, a baby can normally see quite clearly—as far as across the room. Babies usually start to recognize strangers at about six to seven months of age.

A baby's eye colour is genetically determined and does not become permanent until at least nine to twelve months or even longer. Most babies are born with blue eyes, which may darken during their first years. Children can have completely different eye colours from either of their parents.

## Hearing: The First Two Important Years

Babies are able to hear from birth, and will respond to voices and other sounds starting from a very young age. Your baby will make many sounds, such as laughing, squealing, and especially crying. Babbling will progress to baby's first words sometime around twelve months. But it will probably be another year before baby will be able to say two- to three-word sentences. In order for speech to develop normally, a baby must be able to hear. The first two years is the time during which hearing develops in children. It is important for parents to be able to recognize signs of a hearing problem as early as possible and seek medical attention if there are any concerns. Here is a guide of signs of normal hearing development by age through the first two years of life.

### By Four Months of Age a Baby Should

- Move or react when someone speaks or in response to any noise.
- Startle when there is a very loud noise .

### By Seven Months a Baby Should

- Turn his or her head toward a voice or a noise (when a parent calls, even without being seen).
- Stir or move in response to a noise or voice.
- Startle when there is a large sound.

### By Nine Months a Baby Should

- Turn his or her head to find out where a sound is coming from.
- Turn around if a parent is calling from behind.
- Stir or move in response to voice or any sound.
- Startle when there is a very loud noise.

### At Twelve Months a Baby Should

- Turn his or her head in all directions and show interest in a person's voice or a particular sound.
- Repeat sounds that parents make.
- Startle in response to a loud noise.

### At Two Years of Age a Child Should

- Be able to point out a part of his body when asked without seeing the person's lips move.
- Be able to point to the right picture when asked. For example, "Where is the dog? Where is the bird?"
- Be able to do simple tasks like give you one of his or her toys when asked, without seeing your lips move.

If your child does not do these things at the appropriate age as listed above, or if you have any doubts about your child's hearing, speak to your healthcare provider.

## Is There a Special Hearing Test for Babies?

Yes. During a usual hearing test or Audiogram, a sound is played into the child's ear and the child is asked to signal that she heard the sound. Obviously, the younger a child, the more difficult this is. In a baby, the technician looks for signs such as startling—body or facial movements that indicate the sound was heard. However, as one can imagine with babies, this can be quite difficult and quite crude.

Fortunately, there exists a more sophisticated and reliable test called the Auditory Evoked Response Test. Normally, when sound is heard, it passes from the ear as an electrical signal through the auditory (hearing) nerve to the back of the brain where hearing is decoded and understood. By placing small electrodes on the baby's head, the travelling electrical signal can be recorded on a graph. During this test, a sound is played and the response to the sound is then recorded on the graph. If the graph picks up normal electrical activity of the auditory nerve in response to the sound, this is considered normal.

Once a hearing loss (deafness) is confirmed, the child is evaluated by an ENT (Ear, Nose, and Throat) doctor and other specialists whose aim is to attempt to restore the hearing loss through hearing aids or, in some cases, cochlear implants (devices inserted into the child's ear or ears). In any case, the child will also need to have special speech therapy to help her talk and develop language as normally as possible.

## What Exactly Is a Hearing Problem?

When we talk about hearing problems, we really mean deafness—not being able to hear. And there are two types of deafness. One is neurosensory deafness, in which the hearing nerves don't work properly. The other one is conductive hearing loss, which basically we see very commonly in children who get recurrent ear infections whereby the space behind the eardrum is full of fluid that blocks the conduction or transmission of sound. So conductive hearing is not the same as neurosensory deafness. Hearing loss related to recurrent ear infections is usually not permanent and treated differently. I discuss this in more detail in a later section of this book.

### Early Detection Is Important

The earlier a hearing loss is detected the better. Firstly, if the hearing loss can be treated, then it should be, right away. Additionally, the earlier the hearing loss is restored, the quicker the child will start to develop and catch up in terms of speaking and language skills.

### Children at High Risk

There are certain risk factors that we know are associated with hearing difficulties or deafness. These include:

- Premature babies are at higher risk.
- Babies who have been given certain antibiotics (e.g. aminoglycosides such as gentamycin) which are known to be ototoxic, meaning they are toxic to the hearing (auditory) nerve itself.
- Children who have had infections of the central nervous system such as meningitis or encephalitis are also at risk for having hearing difficulties.
- A family history of hereditary deafness: we know there are certain families with what we call congenital neurosensory deafness, in which children are at higher risk of becoming deaf.

## Tooth Development

Most babies will erupt their first teeth between six and eight months old, but it can be normal if the first tooth does not appear before twelve to fourteen months. This varies from baby to baby. Despite the fact that babies are born without any visible teeth, on the inside, tooth development and growth has already begun by the third or fourth month of the pregnancy.

Usually the first tooth that erupts is the lower (mandibular) central incisor, on average at six and a half months of age. The rest of the lower teeth continue to progressively erupt through twenty to thirty months of age in this order: the central incisors are followed by the lateral or side incisors, then the canines, and first and second molars. The upper (maxillary) teeth tend to start a bit later, at about seven and a half months through twenty to thirty months and in the same order as the lower teeth.

It is important to stress that sometimes a baby may have teething symptoms (drooling and irritability) for weeks before teeth actually erupt. This reflects that the teeth are growing and developing inside the gums. Also, I want to stress that, despite many myths that teething causes medical symptoms, there is no evidence that teething causes fever, colds, or diarrhea.

# IMMUNIZATION

Another important preventative health measure is immunization. Your baby's young body is just learning to fight off infection, so it's crucial that your child be vaccinated against a host of childhood illnesses. Immunization is one of the most important steps you can take to ensure your baby's current and future health. Since immunization was first invented, it has saved hundreds of thousands of children's lives. Your child's healthcare provider will discuss the immunization schedule with you and will describe the various vaccines, the diseases they protect your child from, and the possible side effects your child may experience.

## THE CASE FOR VACCINATION

Every year, in developing countries, millions of children less than five years of age die. What is even more shocking is that most of the deaths are due to problems that we in North America do not have to face. For example, these children die of malnutrition and dehydration from diarrhea, because they do not have an adequate food supply nor clean drinking water. Pneumonia, measles, and malaria are also among the top killers. The common trend across these causes is that they are preventable. Agencies like the United Nations and the World Health Organization (WHO) are constantly struggling to provide the basics in all countries, including access to clean water, an adequate and nutritious food supply, vaccination, anti-malaria nets, and medications. Such interventions would literally save millions of lives. Unfortunately, in many countries, these attempts are hampered by local political, civil, and even military unrest.

Reflecting on the above state of affairs, I cannot help but think how lucky we are in North America and other developed parts of the world. Yes, we may have our own health system issues, especially in the US and Canada; however, most childhood infections and their devastating consequences are extremely rare in developed countries. This in large part is due to the availability of clean water, sanitation, and very importantly, vaccination.

Looking at vaccinations through the lens of the developing world is quite eye-opening. Vaccines are probably one of the most significant advances in modern-day medicine. Even in developed or richer countries, when for one reason or another vaccines are not given for a specific disease, that infection rate rises. In Russia, during the 1980s, post the collapse of the iron curtain, political and economic unrest led to a shortage of the diphtheria vaccine. As a result, diphtheria cases began to appear. As soon as the vaccination supply was re-established, diphtheria cases were once again fully prevented. A similar incident occurred in England, when there was widespread media concern about the safety of the vaccine against whooping cough (pertussis). During this time, the number of whooping cough cases increased tremendously. Again, once vaccination rates went up, the cases of whooping cough decreased dramatically. Whooping cough and diphtheria are potentially deadly diseases.

As a pediatrician, I have seen children die of meningitis. I remember one case in particular, when a child died of meningitis due to the bacteria called *Haemophilus Influenzae* (not the flu virus). Tragically, a few weeks later a vaccine for this disease was released. This vaccine would have prevented this deadly infection.

I hope these reflections can help you better understand and appreciate vaccines and their importance. Yes, there may be some rare side effects and we constantly strive to improve vaccines to make them as safe and effective as possible. However, if you or anyone you know thinks of vaccines in a negative way, just think of the millions of children who die annually because they are not vaccinated. After consideration of the above, I hope the terms "vaccine-preventable-disease," "immunization," and "vaccination" ring positive tones. In the next part of this chapter, I will discuss exactly what vaccines are and how they work.

## About Vaccinations

Vaccination (also known as immunization) is a simple procedure involving the use of vaccines that protect children (and adults) from serious and sometimes fatal infectious diseases by strengthening their immunity (their body's ability to fight off these diseases). Babies are born with a degree of natural, inherited immunity, which they acquire during pregnancy from their mothers' blood. That immunity is reinforced during breastfeeding, as breast milk is rich in antibodies, especially in the first few days after birth. But this type of passive, inherited immunity is only temporary; it wears off during the first year of life. This leaves the child vulnerable to a host of serious diseases. But with the help of vaccinations, children can develop protective immunity against these diseases. Vaccines have proven extremely effective in controlling and even eradicating some major childhood diseases. Indeed, smallpox—a severe and often fatal disease that used to be common among children—has been entirely wiped out by worldwide immunization.

### How Do Vaccines Work?

Vaccines are preparations made up of a specific selection of dead or weakened germs (bacteria or viruses), which are administered orally, by injection, or through inhalation. When living disease organisms enter a person's system, the body fights infection by producing antibodies that attack and kill the organisms. In a similar fashion, when these dead or weakened germs contained in vaccines enter a person's system, the body responds by producing antibodies that attack and kill the organisms without causing the serious symptoms that occur during the real infection. So when, or if ever, the real bacteria or virus enters the body, it already has antibodies ready to immediately protect against that particular infection. As a result, the body develops immunity to that particular disease, and is protected for months, years, or a lifetime, depending on the vaccine. Some vaccines induce prolonged or even lifelong immunity to certain diseases, and can be given just once. But others, such as pertussis and diphtheria, only induce a temporary immunity. These vaccines require repeat injections (called boosters) in order to maintain protection against such diseases.

## Are Vaccines Safe?

Generally, vaccines are safe and very effective. The benefits of immunization far outweigh any risks. Typical side effects may include a mild fever, local redness, and swelling at the site of the needle injection, or a slight rash, depending on the vaccine. More serious side effects are rare. Your child's healthcare provider may recommend acetaminophen to treat or prevent fever and local injection pain or redness, and will explain exactly what to look for after each vaccine administration. Again, I stress that almost all children receiving vaccines have minimal or no side effects.

## Keeping an Immunization Record

It's a good idea to keep a record of immunizations received for each person in the family. Record sheets or booklets are usually provided for this purpose. In some counties, there are apps or online tools designed to record vaccinations. They are valuable if your family moves countries or changes healthcare providers, and are a handy reminder of upcoming vaccines or boosters. The record is also proof of your child's protection against certain infectious diseases; proof which you may need to enroll your child in school or travel overseas. Your child's immunization record should specify the type of vaccine, and be dated and signed by your healthcare provider each time an immunization is given. The record should be kept at home in a safe, accessible place, and should be taken with the family on trips away from home.

## Available Vaccines

Although each country may differ slightly for the requirement, timing, and doses of particular vaccines, most countries seek to prevent the same diseases. Vaccination against these diseases is mostly required during the first eighteen months of life. Also, new bioscientific techniques now allow for the development of new or more effective vaccines. It is a good idea to discuss any newly available vaccine with your healthcare provider to see whether your child may benefit from it.

For the first eighteen months, here is a list of available vaccines and the diseases (infections) they prevent:

- Diphtheria;
- *Haemophilus Influenzae* type b (Hib);
- Hepatitis;
- Influenza (flu);
- Measles;
- Meningitis (Meningococcal Disease);
- Mumps;
- Pertussis (also known as Whooping Cough);
- Pneumococcal Disease;
- Polio;
- Rotavirus;
- Rubella (also known as German measles);
- Tetanus (also known as Lockjaw);
- Varicella (also known as Chickenpox).

To obtain the schedule for your baby's immunizations and more specific details about vaccines, their potential side effects and the diseases they prevent, consult your healthcare provider and refer to your country's national immunization recommendations and schedule.

# Common Baby and Childcare Issues

In this section of my book, I have compiled information and facts that reflect frequently asked questions by parents of newborns and young children. I think that this section will help you be better prepared and understand what to expect around some of the common baby and childcare issues. In addition, I hope it will help you to recognize what is normal and what is not. Note that this is a very general listing and description of the common issues. Your healthcare provider will supply you with more detailed and specific information.

## Biting

Children biting other children is a rather common problem, especially with young children during the first few years of their lives. In fact, according to the National Association for the Education of Young Children, one out of ten toddlers bites and there are four different types of biters.

### The Experimental Biter

An infant or young child may take an experimental bite out of a mother's breast or a caregiver's shoulder. Experimental biters may simply want to touch, smell, and taste others in order to learn. In other words, they need to experiment. This type of biting may also be a result of teething pain.

## The Frustrated Biter

Some children may not yet have the skills to deal with wanting an adult's attention or another child's toy. Even though the child may not intend to harm, they may bite; parents and caregivers need to react with disapproval and watch for signs of rising frustration and give positive reinforcement when a child communicates effectively, without biting.

## The Threatened Biter

Certain children bite in self-defence, because they are overwhelmed or afraid in their surroundings, and bite as a means of regaining control. Situations such as newly separated parents, the death of a grandparent, or a mother returning to work may be stressing or threatening the child.

## The Power Biter

Some children experience a strong need for autonomy and control. As soon as they see the response they get from biting, this behaviour is strongly reinforced, so they continue to bite. In this situation, the biter should be given choices throughout the day. Also, they need a lot of positive reinforcement when they do things like sharing and saying thanks, instead of resorting to biting. If the biter gets attention when not biting, she or he will not have to bite in order to gain as a sense of power.

Here are some general rules adapted from the National Association for the Education of Young Children on how to approach children who bite others:

- If a child bites, remain calm and in control.
- Never hit or bite back a child for biting.
- Parents and caregivers need to cooperate and ensure the same approach is used in all settings
- Be ready to intervene immediately,
- And teach children how to control themselves, something that encourages the development of confidence and self-esteem.

**Be aware** that it is important to ensure that any area that is bitten is cleaned immediately and seek medical attention if the skin is broken. Human bites can transmit dangerous bacteria from the mouth to the damaged skin area and cause severe infections. This can be prevented by appropriate cleaning of the wound and in many cases, by using antibiotics.

## Breast Engorgement

Many newborn babies—both boys and girls—seem to have swollen breasts. They may even have a milky discharge from their nipples. This is normal and caused by mother's female hormones that cross the placenta just before birth. They will disappear within a few weeks. In the meantime, don't try to squeeze any discharge from the breasts, because this can irritate them or cause infection.

# Constipation in Babies

Many babies and young children are constipated at times. Parents might suspect iron in the formula of bottle-fed babies, but research has shown that iron in a milk formula does not cause constipation. As a matter of fact, parents frequently consult with this problem. It may be normal for babies to have infrequent bowel movements. The regularity and frequency of bowel movements varies from one baby to another, and can even change in the same baby from day to day. The stool frequency in breastfed babies can vary even more; for example from eight to twelve bowel movements per day to one bowel movement every few days. A baby's stool is initially quite liquid, especially in breastfed babies. As a child gets older, the stool becomes more formed or pasty, often corresponding with the time of starting solids. A baby is considered to be truly constipated only if the bowel movements are hard, painful, and/or associated with signs of discomfort, such as abdominal pain or crying while passing a stool. If this is the case, consult your healthcare provider.

Generally, once a constipated baby has been evaluated and all is found to be normal, the problem can be treated simply by giving your child more liquid or by adding some table sugar to the child's milk. You should discuss this with your healthcare provider. Most of the time, this will be enough.

Remember, laxatives should not be given to young children.

## Crying and Colic

In the past, I would spend a lot of time discussing colic with parents. Basically, the classic definition of colic is really a description of the frequency of crying.

Traditionally, colic is defined as continual or persistent crying without any apparent reason, typically lasting more than three hours per day, more than three days per week for at least three weeks. It usually begins at around two or three weeks of age, and subsides on its own by twelve weeks.

Babies with colic were described as having prolonged bouts of intense, high-pitched crying. Some infants draw their legs up and clench their fists, as if in pain. Spells of crying tend to occur at around the same time each day, often in the early evening. Babies with colic may be inconsolable; nothing their parents do seems to soothe them. In spite of persistent crying, these babies do not have any apparent symptoms of illness.

However, when we now look at the latest studies on babies' crying habits, as described in a previous section of this book, we realize that colic and the PURPLE period of crying are really the same.

Actually, these classic colic symptoms exactly describe the acronym PURPLE.

- **P: Peak of Crying**—Baby may cry more each week. They tend to cry more at two months and then less at three to five months.
- **U: Unexpected**—Crying can come and go, and you do not know why.
- **R: Resists Soothing**—Baby may not stop crying, no matter what you try.
- **P: Painlike Face**—A crying baby may look like they are in pain, even when they are not.

- **L: Long-Lasting**—Crying can last as much as five hours a day, or more.
- **E: Evening**—Baby may cry more during the late afternoon or evening. I refer to this as a crying shift.

During the PURPLE period of crying, parents may be relieved to find out that, however alarming the bouts of crying are, the crying itself is not a serious condition. Though these babies may appear to be in distress, they are usually in good health and are growing and developing normally. Parents should be certain, however, that the baby does not suffer from any other medical conditions that could be producing the crying. If bouts of crying are accompanied by vomiting, abdominal bloating, fever, or other signs of illness seek medical attention immediately.

The best way to approach and deal with an excessively crying baby is to assess and monitor its effect on the parents or child caregivers. During the first few months of life, we know that some babies will cry more intensely than others will; but all babies cry. If a parent is frustrated or tired, then the crying is indeed a problem. If on the other hand, despite the crying, both the baby and parents are content and happy—this is great!

Although intense or excessive crying is not a serious medical problem, it can cause a great deal of stress and anxiety within the family. Excessive crying can wear on everybody's nerves, and can lead to feelings of parental inadequacy and constant worry. This kind of anxiety isn't good for either the parents or the baby. It is important never to shake a crying baby out of frustration or anger. The crying is neither the parents' nor the baby's fault. Parents who are feeling stressed or burned out should seek relief for themselves whenever possible. They should leave the baby in the hands of a competent babysitter, and take time out for a movie, a dinner out, or just a few hours of quiet relaxation. Taking frequent breaks can go a long way toward helping parents cope with their baby's crying.

# Dental Care

## Teething

Teething pain may be soothed by giving the baby a cool teething ring or washcloth to suck on. Local anesthetic freezing creams—available over the counter at pharmacies—should not be used in children. Sometimes, giving your baby acetaminophen drops orally may help with the pain. Your healthcare provider or pharmacist can provide you with the correct dosage and specific instructions.

## Dental Care and Oral Hygiene

Oral hygiene and care is essential. As soon as teeth develop, they should be cleaned daily with a wet gauze or washcloth **without** toothpaste. Once all the teeth grow in, parents can switch to using a toothbrush, but they should not use toothpaste until the child is old enough to understand not to swallow it. Do not use toothpaste for children under three years of age unless told to do so by your dentist.

For children aged three to six, use toothpaste sparingly on the toothbrush—the size of a pea and no larger. Review proper tooth brushing techniques for your child with your dentist, and be sure that your child can brush properly before allowing him or her to brush on their own.

As long as the spaces between the teeth are wide enough to allow the toothbrush access, flossing is not necessary. As soon as the spaces between the teeth are tight enough to allow it, regular daily flossing should also begin.

## Prevention of Dental Caries (Cavities)

Dental caries (better known as cavities) are seen frequently, but thanks to better preventative measures, there has been a decrease in their numbers over the last twenty years. Despite the decreasing trend, the current rate of caries in children is still high. According to the CDC, more than 25 percent of two- to five-year-olds have one or more cavities. Aside from causing the child local pain and an infection that can sometimes spread to the eye and brain, we now know that dental caries and poor dental hygiene are also linked to higher rates of chronic diseases such as diabetes and heart conditions. So proper oral hygiene is not just for the sake of the teeth, mouth, and gums; it contributes to overall health and wellness.

One of the most important factors related to cavities is the consumption of carbohydrates or sugar. Actually, the development of dental caries depends more on how often a child consumes sugary foods rather than the exact amount. In babies and infants who still drink from the bottle, one of the most important causes of caries is putting them to bed with a bottle. Both juice and milk contain sugar, which remains on the baby's teeth overnight, resulting in Nursing Bottle Caries, usually among the upper teeth. Aside from the pain and discomfort of the cavities, the treatment itself can also be painful and, in extreme cases, the baby teeth need to be extracted. In young children, this may require heavy sedation or even a general anesthetic. Clearly, the goal is to prevent cavities in children. Modifying the diet to decrease the frequency of sugar consumption is very important. Again, I stress that bottle-fed children should never be put to bed with the bottle.

Aside from the oral hygiene precautions described above, fluoride, a substance found naturally in ground water in some geographic locations, is another effective measure against dental caries. Babies and young children may need additional supplementation of fluoride, depending on their age and the level of fluoride in your local drinking water, either added by your municipality or present naturally. Your local municipality can tell you the amount of fluoride in your drinking water. Knowing this, your healthcare provider can then decide if supplementation is needed and how much. This is important, as we do not want to give too much fluoride to babies and young children. For the same reason, when brushing teeth in children aged three to six, toothpaste containing fluoride should be put sparingly on the toothbrush … the size of a pea and no larger. Again, we want to avoid excessive fluoride ingestion.

I believe that community water fluoridation is one of the greatest public health achievements of the 20th century, and I am not alone in this assertion. More than ninety national and international health organizations, including Health Canada, the Canadian Dental Association, the Canadian Medical Association, the US Centers for Disease Control and Prevention, and the World Health Organization, endorse the use of fluoride at recommended levels to prevent tooth decay. Many major scientific studies have also concluded that community water fluoridation is a safe and effective method of reducing tooth decay at all stages of life, and that there is no credible scientific evidence to suggest adverse health effects related to water fluoridation.

## When Should Baby Visit the Dentist?

The American Academy of Pediatric Dentistry currently recommends that the first dental visit be scheduled for six months *after* the first tooth erupts or at one year of age, whichever comes first. This gives the dentist the opportunity to examine for existing problems and caries, assess overall oral hygiene and health, and look for any abnormalities in tooth development. In general, the first visit is a get-to-know-one-another visit. Obviously, if there is an injury to the teeth or if there are signs of discoloration or tooth decay, a pediatric dentist should be seen earlier.

# Diaper Area Care

## Diaper Rash

Diaper rash, which is referred to as diaper dermatitis, is caused by prolonged exposure to wet or soiled diapers. The urine's wet consistency causes the skin to be tender and become irritated or inflamed. Diaper rash can occur with snug fitting diapers, either disposable or cloth. While most babies develop diaper rash at some time, especially during the first ten months, the rash occurs less often in breastfed babies. Fortunately, diaper rash is usually not a serious problem.

Factors that may contribute to diaper rash or dermatitis include:

- Wet and dirty diapers;
- Diarrhea, because it is acidic and tends to burn or irritate the skin around the anus and buttocks;
- The acidic content of solids foods;
- Coloured diapers; the dye itself may irritate a child's bottom;
- A fungal or yeast infection caused by Candida , which can occur after a baby has taken antibiotics.

## How is Diaper Rash Treated?

Once a rash develops, the goal is to keep the area clean and protected. This is achieved by:

- Changing the diaper as soon as possible after a bowel movement and cleaning the area with a soft cloth and warm water, rinsing and drying it well;
- Using barrier creams applied to the skin in the diaper area. These creams or ointments serve to protect the already irritated skin.

- In severe cases of diaper dermatitis, a special cream or ointment containing a small amount of hydrocortisone may be necessary. A healthcare provider can easily assess whether or not such a treatment is needed.

## About Candidal Diaper Rash

*Candida* is a fungus that can cause infections of the skin. When this fungus infects the skin in the diaper areas, it is called a Candidal diaper rash. The rash tends to occur in the creases, in the groin, in the skin folds, and buttocks, and is usually very red with smaller spots called satellite lesions. There are usually no other associated signs or symptoms. The rash is painless and is not itchy. A doctor can easily recognize this type of rash. The treatment of Candidal diaper rash is the application of a prescribed cream containing an anti-fungal medication. This cream should be applied during diaper changes, after washing the area with mild soap and warm water, and drying it. To avoid spread of *Candida* to others, parents should wash their hands carefully after the diaper change. This rash starts to go away within a few days after starting the treatment.

## Diaper Rash Prevention

Here are some tips on how to prevent diaper rash:

- Change your baby's wet diaper frequently.
- Keep your baby out of a diaper for short periods to allow the skin to dry.
- Avoid coloured diapers.
- Make sure that the diaper and plastic pants are not so tight as to exclude air from circulating inside the diaper.

If you think your child has a *Candida* infection, contact your health-care provider.

To protect against diaper rash, you may want to apply a barrier cream.

## Earwax

Wax is part of the ear's natural protection, its defence against germs and other particles.

Practically speaking, earwax is not bad. The main difficulty is that the wax can completely cover the eardrum. In very rare cases, the wax can build up so much that it can actually block hearing. Contrary to popular belief, wax buildup does not cause ear infections or any other serious problems. What can happen is that when a doctor examines the ear, he or she might be unable to see the eardrum and, therefore, would be unable to determine if there is an infection or other problem.

### Tips on Cleaning Your Child's Earwax at Home

**Never insert** Q-tips or any other long objects into a child's ear.

- When bathing a young child, gently wash around the outside of the ear with a wet washcloth.
- If a child tends to have a lot of wax, place a few drops of mineral or baby oil in the ear and cover it with a cotton plug overnight. Doing this once or twice will usually clean out the wax completely.
- Commercially available drops called cerumenolytic agents designed to melt or break down the wax are not recommended, as they tend to irritate the ear canal.

### What if Earwax Cannot Be Removed At Home?

In this case, the wax should be removed by a healthcare professional. There are two ways this can be done.

### Syringing the Ear

While the child is lying down, a syringe full of warm water is gently inserted into the ear and the water is flushed into the canal removing or washing out the wax. It may take a few tries before the wax is fully removed.

### Curetting

A thin instrument called a curette, held like a pencil, is used to directly remove or literally pick out the wax. Under direct visualization with a light, the provider gently removes the wax using the curette.

Generally, these techniques are not painful, but obviously will be more difficult to perform in younger children. If the wax is very hard, however, sometimes the parents will be asked to apply oil or hydrogen peroxide drops beforehand, in order to soften the wax.

# Foot and Leg Issues

Many parents worry about their baby's lower limbs, because they may not look straight or aligned. During the first few years of life, the shape and look of the legs and feet may change. Whenever we think about lower limb issues, we need to think of the three main parts of the legs: the hips, knees, and feet. In this chapter, I will review some of the common issues about babies' lower extremities, many of which are normal or variants of normal for a baby's stage of development.

## Hips

During baby's first and subsequent physical examinations, the assessment of the hips is important. This is to ensure that the hips are not dislocated. Congenital or developmental dislocation of the hip occurs in up to 2 percent of newborns. By moving the legs in certain ways while feeling the hip joint area for a clicking noise, the healthcare provider can make the diagnosis. Once there is a suspicion of hip dislocation, X-rays may be needed and the child will be evaluated by a pediatric orthopedic surgeon. The treatment is usually the placement of the hips in a harness or cast, usually for four to six weeks, depending on the individual situation. Left untreated, congenital hip dislocation can result in long-term consequences such as walking problems and arthritis.

## Knees

During the first two years of life, normal babies are bowlegged, in other words, their knees are far from each other. This is referred to as *genu varum* and is normal.

Between their third and fourth years, children's knees start to curve inwards to touch each other, or become knock-knees (*genu valgum*). After this, the knees return to a position somewhere in the middle.

Again, this is part of normal leg development. As children get older and if knock knees persist and are significant, they can be evaluated by an orthopedic surgeon.

## In-Toeing and Out-Toeing

"In-toeing" is when the leg or foot points inward and "out-toeing" is when the leg or foot points outward. Both are common in babies and young children. These foot rotational concerns almost always go away on their own without any future significant walking or related problems. When we evaluate these children, we look at the three possible sources: the hip, the knees, and the feet. The approach and treatment, if any, will vary depending on the source, the location, and the nature of the cause. In very rare cases, if the rotation persists beyond eight years of age and is associated with foot pain or walking difficulties, surgical repair may be required. Reassuringly, however, the vast majority of these foot-rotations go away spontaneously.

Note that it is not uncommon for toddlers to tiptoe when they first walk. As long as there are no ankle issues (they are very rare), tiptoeing is considered normal.

## Shoes

Parents often worry that they need to buy special shoes for their infants or toddlers. Actually, babies do not need footwear to start walking. The only reason we put shoes on children is to protect their feet and avoid slipping. Children who grow up without shoes learn to walk just as well as children who wear shoes. So there is no need for getting special so-called orthopedic shoes, as long as the shoe provides good support and protects the baby's feet.

# Genital Area Care

## Newborn Baby Girls

### Vaginal Discharge and Bleeding and Swollen Genitals

In newborn girls, there's often a clear or whitish vaginal discharge that may be tinged with blood. The genital area may also be swollen. These features are perfectly normal, and are caused by mother's female hormones that cross the placenta just before birth. They will disappear within a few weeks.

## Newborn Baby Boys

### Penis Care

If your baby boy has not been circumcised, his penis requires no special care. Do not try to pull back his foreskin to clean it.

Although recent studies have shown some health benefits to circumcision, experts state that the decision is a parental one based on personal or religious beliefs or practices. If you decide to have your baby boy circumcised, the only recommendation I have is to ensure that all necessary and appropriate measures are taken to control the pain during the procedure.

If your child has been circumcised, his penis will be wrapped in gauze after the operation. Each time you change his diaper, apply fresh gauze dabbed in petroleum jelly or some other ointment, until the penis is fully healed. It's also important to keep the penis as dry as possible during this time. Once the incision has healed, simply wash the penis with soap and water.

## Hydrocele In Boys

A hydrocele is a collection of fluid in the scrotum. Usually one can easily feel the testes separately in a baby's scrotum. With fluid in it, the scrotum feels full and one cannot feel the testes. During a physical examination of a baby boy with hydrocele, when a healthcare provider shines a light on the scrotum, he or she can see the light shine through it, indicating that fluid is present. This fluid is a remnant or remains of the prenatal scrotal sac and testicular formation; it usually goes away on its own within a few months. If a hydrocele persists or has an associated hernia, then a small operation may be needed.

## Undescended Testicles

The testicles (testes) are formed in the baby's abdomen during the pregnancy and by the time of delivery, they have travelled down into the scrotum. However, in about 5 percent of babies, one or both of the testes cannot be felt in the scrotum during a routine physical examination. This is called an undescended testicle, also known as cryptorchidism, when it is stuck en route to the scrotum or is still in the abdomen. Usually, only one of the testes is affected and it is more common in boys born prematurely. In most situations, the testicle descends by six months of age. However, if by this time it still has not descended, the baby is usually referred to a specialist for a surgery called an orchidopexy. This is a short operation done under a general anesthetic in a day surgery setting.

The reason for concern with undescended testicles is because there is an increased risk of infertility and also testicular cancer if the testicle remains in the abdomen.

Sometimes in babies where the testes have descended normally, it may be difficult to feel them in the scrotum. This is because there is a reflex that pulls the testes up when the leg or groin area is touched. It is referred to as retractile testes and they are not considered undescended. In such cases, I ask parents to examine the baby while he is in a warm bath. Under these conditions, the testicles are usually in the scrotum.

# Head, Neck, and Related Concerns

## Head

### Cephalohematomas and Head Moulding

A cephalohematoma looks like a swollen bruise on the scalp of a newborn baby and is quite common. It is caused by the pressure of the physical pushing of the birth process itself, especially if a vacuum is used to assist. Similarly, forceps used for a difficult delivery may cause bruises on the scalp and on the face of a newborn baby. Cephalohematomas and facial bruising do not usually cause any serious problems, except for an increased risk of jaundice. Usually, a cephalohematoma goes away on its own within a few weeks or months, without any treatment being needed.

Also, sometimes the head of a newborn baby seems to be oddly shaped, oblong, or pointed like a cone. This is referred to as moulding and is the result of pressure on the head and skull during the birth. Remember that the skull is made up of a few bones that are not connected or fused yet. So any pressure from travelling through the birth canal during labour and delivery will shape and mould the skull differently. Moulding usually resolves on its own without any long-term consequences.

### Positional Plagiocephaly

The term "plagiocephaly" refers to a flat area or spot on the head. Because a newborn's skull is made up of a few bones that can move, its shape can be altered or affected if the baby is in a certain position for long periods of time. So if the head has a flat spot due to a certain constant position, it is referred to as Positional Plagiocephaly. As a result of the recommendation to put infants on their backs to sleep in order to prevent Sudden Infant Death Syndrome (SIDS), there has been an increase in the rate of positional plagiocephaly. A 2013 study estimates the incidence of positional plagiocephaly is at more than 45 percent of infants aged seven to twelve weeks old. In most situations, there are no long-term effects, except perhaps for some cosmetic ones. In severe cases, a neurosurgeon may be consulted to assess the child's brain and skull growth and development.

### Prevention of Positional Plagiocephaly

Plagiocephaly progression can be stopped and ideally prevented in the first place.

Here are some tips to help prevent positional plagiocephaly adapted from the American Academy of Pediatrics:

- Beginning at birth, during sleep, nightly switch the direction your baby faces while lying on his back: one night facing toward the left and the next toward the right, and so on.
- While awake and being observed, your baby should spend time in the prone position (tummy time) on a firm surface for at least thirty to sixty minutes per day.
- Do not place baby for long periods of time indoors in car safety seats and swings or in other seating that puts them on their backs. Do not put them in places that cause constant pressure on the back of the heads.

The incidence of positional plagiocephaly peaks at four months and starts to improve significantly by six months of age. Once a flat area or spot has developed, the above preventive strategies may be used as well as the following:

- Position the infant so that the rounded side of the head is placed against the mattress and the flat side is not.
- Where applicable, change the location of the crib in the room so that the baby will need to look away from the flat side to see her parents and others in her room.

In general, most infants improve if the above measures are followed for two to three months. In severe cases of deformity or for the babies who do not improve after six months of age, special helmets that mould the head may be an option.

### Cradle Cap

During the first two or three months of life, some babies develop yellow-red scales or crusts on the scalp called Cradle Cap. The scales and crusting can also occur behind the ears, on the eyebrows, and tend to resolve on their own by one year of age. Cradle cap does not hurt the baby and can be treated at home quite simply. After each bath, soften the crusty scales by applying baby oil. Then gently comb your baby's hair forward and downward using a comb or soft brush to loosen the scales. Difficult areas can be treated with a washcloth or cotton ball dipped in oil to remove scales and then rinsed out.

### Hair Falling Out

Some parents really worry when they start to see their baby's hair begin to fall out between three and four months of age. It is perfectly normal for a baby to lose their hair, as the newborn hair is being shed to allow new hair to grow in.

## Tongue-tie

Tongue-tie or Ankyloglossia refers to a short frenulum (also known as a frenum), which is the piece of skin (a ligament) that connects the bottom of the tongue to the floor of the mouth. Theoretically, if the frenulum is short, there may be difficulty speaking, nursing, or feeding. In the past, because of this fear, short frenulums were cut at birth. We now understand that tongue-tie really has no effect on speech. A simple test to screen whether or not there may be a problem with tongue-tie is to ask the child to stick out the tip of the tongue to touch the upper lip. If this can be done there usually is no associated problem and no reason for any treatment. Even if the tongue cannot fully touch the upper lip, if the function is normal (normal speech and feeding), then there is no treatment.

Very rarely, if the frenulum is very short and really prevents the tongue from moving and functioning normally, it is cut surgically. This is particularly important if the tongue-tie is causing breastfeeding difficulties. Although tongue-tie tends not to interfere with bottle feeding, it is a recognized possible cause of breastfeeding problems. If a baby with tongue-tie has a poor latch or a poor suck, and is unable to drink enough at the breast, cutting the frenulum will likely solve the problem. This of course applies only if the tongue-tie is found to be the cause. Your healthcare provider or nearest breastfeeding support group can provide you with additional specific information.

## Blocked Tear Duct

A baby with a blocked tear duct (also known as a lacrimal duct) presents with a constantly runny (teary) eye. This is usually noticed during the first few weeks of life. The initial treatment is to massage the area between the nose and eye gently and this may open up the ducts. If this fails then a probe procedure is needed. Under general anesthesia, a tiny probe (a tiny iron rod) is placed in the tear duct opening to stretch it or unblock it. The procedure will, I am sure, be explained to you in great detail by your ophthalmologist.

## Torticollis

Torticollis, also known as wryneck or twisted neck, is seen commonly in newborn babies and infants up to three months of age. Although we do not know the exact cause of torticollis, it is believed to be related to the position of the head and neck in the uterus during pregnancy. This position puts pressure on a major neck muscle on one side and baby is born with the affected side more contracted or shorter than the other. As a result, the baby will then tend to tilt her head toward the side where the muscle is shorter or more tightened. Some babies with torticollis may develop positional plagiocephaly on one side, due to lying in one position all the time.

Most babies get better through stretching exercises. Once your baby is evaluated for this, your healthcare provider will recommend and describe neck-stretching exercises you can do at home during each diaper change. In general, it takes up to six months or more to resolve. Sometimes, the baby will be referred to a physiotherapist for evaluation and additional exercises depending on the individual situation. If your baby's torticollis is not improving with the stretching exercises, please speak with your healthcare provider.

# Humidifier Use

Parents often wonder about the need for humidifiers at home and what type is best. We need to have a certain level of humidity in the air we breathe in through our nose. The normal or ideal indoor humidity level is about 40 percent to 45 percent. Humidity levels over 45 percent can indeed be harmful, both directly and indirectly.

In asthmatic children, for example, high humidity may make the asthma symptoms worse. Indirectly, high humidity affects our health adversely by promoting mould growth and dust mites. Dust mites are microscopic insects that live in dust found in upholstered furniture and they thrive on high humidity. Dust mites are considered to be very significant irritants in asthma and in chronic nasal allergies. Moulds grow in the presence of high humidity and have been associated with causing or worsening asthma and other respiratory symptoms as well as other health problems.

How can you determine what the level of humidity is in your house? Special hygrometers, which look like thermometers, are readily available at any hardware or department store. These instruments can help parents monitor the humidity level at home.

Under normal conditions, and if the humidity levels are normal, a humidifier is not necessary. On the other hand, in the presence of high humidity (over 45 percent), and especially if a child has chronic asthma and/or respiratory allergies, the humidity needs to be decreased by using a dehumidifier.

Low humidity is not good either as it dries up the respiratory tract, including the nose. In the case of low humidity, a central humidifier may help to bring up the humidity and maintain it at normal levels.

Well, the issue can get even more complicated. We know that one of the treatments of a cold is humidity, because it helps the congested child breathe more easily. So, in this case, extra humidification for a short time may help, even if the humidity level in the room is normal. However, I do not generally recommend extra humidification even during a cold in asthmatic children. Although humidifiers may help a child with a cold, they should not routinely be used in asthmatic children, unless discussed with your healthcare provider.

Presuming that one uses a humidifier, there are several issues. One is cold mist versus warm. I prefer cold, as it is safer. Warm mists may accidentally spill and scald a child. Next, vaporizer versus humidifier? In general, I do not think there is much difference between the two.

What about adding menthol (lotion or rub) to vaporizers? I do not recommend this as some studies have suggested that the associated fumes may be potentially toxic. On a final note, a potential problem relates to not cleaning the filters frequently or adequately. Moisture left in the humidifier (or vaporizer) can harbour moulds and bacteria. An improperly maintained or unclean humidifier may be actually spreading germs and harming a child.

# Infection Prevention

Childhood infections such as the flu and the common cold are caused by germs called viruses, which spread very easily, especially in pre-school and school-age children. Germs can spread from person to person in the following ways:

- Direct hand-to-hand contact or touch.
- Indirect contact; for example if a child touches an infected surface like a toy or a door handle and then puts her hand to her own eyes, nose, or mouth.
- Virus droplets being passed through the air; for example, from coughing and sneezing.

## Preventing Spread of Infection Is Crucial

As there usually is no specific treatment for these infections, the best bet is preventing them in the first place by practising and teaching good infection control and prevention habits.

The following will help prevent germs from spreading to others:

- Children should be taught at an early age to wash their hands after any contact with their mouth and nose, especially before and after meals and snacks.
- Children should be taught to cover their mouth and nose when coughing and sneezing.
- Facial tissues should be used for runny noses and to catch sneezes. These should be immediately put into the garbage after each use.
- Avoid kissing your child on or around the mouth or face.

- Anyone who comes in close contact with someone with the flu should wash their hands before and after contact.
- Dishes and utensils should be washed in hot, soapy water or in the dishwasher.
- Children should not share pacifiers, cups, utensils, washcloths, towels, and toothbrushes.
- Disposable paper cups should be used in the bathroom and kitchen.
- Disinfecting is important as certain germs can live for more than thirty minutes on doorknobs, toilet handles, countertops, and even on toys. Use a disinfectant or soap and hot water to keep these areas and items clean.
- Children should learn at an early age to get used to the good habit of always washing their hands after going to the bathroom.
- Parents and other caregivers should always wash their hands after changing a baby's diaper.

## Jaundice of the Newborn

Jaundice, technically known as hyperbilirubinemia, is seen quite commonly in newborn babies. It is the yellow colour of the skin and whites of the eyes caused by excess bilirubin in the blood. Bilirubin is produced by the normal breakdown of red blood cells, which is collected and cleared by the liver and then transferred to the intestines. In fact, it is the bilirubin in the intestines that darkens the colour of stool. However, during the newborn period, the bilirubin accumulates in the blood temporarily at higher levels than usual. The reason for this accumulation is that the baby's immature liver is overwhelmed by the breakdown of the red blood cells, which are higher in number in a newborn as compared with adults. So the bilirubin from broken down, excess baby red blood cells is an extra load that a newborn baby's liver can't handle. As a result, the blood bilirubin levels are higher. Referred to as physiological jaundice, this occurs in most newborns, usually by the second to the fourth day. It is mild and resolves on its own by the first or second week of age. In addition to physiological or normal jaundice of the newborn, there are various conditions or situations that are associated with jaundice.

- **Jaundice in premature babies:** Because premature babies' livers are even more immature than full-term babies' are, they have an even harder time in clearing the excess bilirubin load at birth. As a result, babies born prematurely (at less than thirty-five weeks of pregnancy) are at higher risk for developing jaundice during the first few days of life.
- **Blood group mismatch:** If a baby has a different blood type from his mother, the mother might produce antibodies that attack and break down the baby's red blood cells. This adds to

the bilirubin load on the baby's liver and results in higher levels of jaundice. This is why mother's blood type is tested during pregnancy. If mother's blood type indicates a potential mismatch or incompatibility, there are some preventive measures that can be taken before a baby is born. Newborn babies with a potential or known mismatch are observed and monitored very carefully as they are at an increased risk for developing dangerously high levels of bilirubin.

- **Breast milk jaundice:** In a very small percentage of breastfed babies, certain substances in breast milk can cause the bilirubin level to rise.
- **Less common cases:** In less common cases, jaundice may indicate another condition such as an infection or even be prolonged or exaggerated by the presence of bruising or cephalohematomas (bruising of the head during child birth).

Although in the vast majority of babies jaundice resolves on its own, levels of bilirubin higher than 25 milligram per decilitre may cause deafness or brain damage. Because of the potential of these rare yet serious complications, all newborn babies are screened and examined for jaundice within a few days of birth.

If you notice your baby's skin or eyes turning yellow or the colour deepens or worsens, seek medical attention. Your healthcare provider will examine the baby and test for bilirubin. Testing for bilirubin levels involves a simple blood test.

## Treating Newborn Jaundice

In most babies, jaundice will go away on its own. If your baby's jaundice seems to be worsened by breastfeeding, speak to your healthcare provider to discuss options that are best suited for your situation.

If the bilirubin level is high, a baby will be tested regularly until the bilirubin starts to drop off to normal levels in the blood. In some cases, this may require readmission to hospital. Some babies with high levels of jaundice, depending on their age and other circumstances, may require phototherapy or light therapy. This involves exposing a baby's skin to special lights, which help speed up the clearance of the bilirubin from the blood. In rare cases, a blood exchange transfusion is used to remove the excess bilirubin from the baby's blood.

# Nasal Congestion

Babies and young children with colds and associated nasal congestion and secretions have a particularly hard time breathing as they are obligate nose breathers. In other words, they don't really know how to breathe through their mouths if their noses are blocked. As they get older, they learn to mouth-breath, and, therefore, become less uncomfortable when their nose is congested. Another important fact is that most younger children do not know how to blow their noses.

## Treatment

As a general rule, cough and/or decongestant syrups and preparations should not be given to children younger than six years of age because of their potential side effects. On the other hand, if a young child is uncomfortable, parents want to help. Most of the time, some simple techniques can be helpful while still avoiding the use of medications.

Here are some practical tips on how to handle a young child's nasal congestion and secretions during a cold:

- Make sure there is adequate humidity in the child's room (40 percent to 45 percent).
- Ensure that the child is drinking enough. An ill child will probably drink less per feed than usual, but will drink more frequently.
- Try to help clear the secretions in the nose. Salt (saline) water drops are helpful, but only if used properly. Just putting a few drops into the nose will not clear out the secretions. Put in the salt water drops and, a minute or two later, use a nasal pump to help suck out and clear the secretions. In this way, you can help the child blow or clean out his nose. This is an important point, because the drops will not directly help clear the secretions. In

fact, what they do is help loosen the dry secretions so that the nasal suction pump can help clear them. Trying to suck out dry secretions with the nasal pump is not very effective. If after these steps a child is still uncomfortable, parents should discuss the next step with their doctor.

As children get older, two things occur: the nasal passages get bigger and are less easily blocked; and children eventually learn to blow their noses on their own. Encouraging them to learn to do this as early as possible is helpful. Often children learn to blow their nose by imitating their parents who are blowing their own noses. Older children who understand the concept of blowing up a balloon or blowing into a straw can be instructed to blow in the same way through their nose. By practising this, they will eventually learn to blow their noses on their own.

## Pacifier Use

All babies are born with the instinct to suck. Sucking a pacifier, a thumb, or a finger is common and has a soothing effect on babies.

Some children don't suck their thumbs; instead, they rely on a pacifier. Pacifier use in babies does not cause any medical or psychological problems. If your baby wants to suck beyond what nursing or bottle-feeding provides, a pacifier will satisfy that need.

**Remember:** pacifiers should not replace or delay meals. Offer a pacifier only after or between feedings, in other words, when your baby is not hungry.

Some babies use a pacifier to fall asleep. The trouble is they often wake up crying for the pacifier when it falls out of their mouths, because they are not able to search out the pacifier themselves. This can be avoided by not getting baby used to falling asleep with a pacifier. Although pacifiers may be soothing, a baby who gets used to falling asleep with a pacifier will have trouble settling down without one. If a baby falls asleep in your arms with a pacifier, remove it before putting baby to bed.

### Pacifier Safety Tips

If your child does take to a pacifier, be sure to provide one that is safe. When buying and using a pacifier, the American Academy of Paediatrics recommends the following:

- Use a one-piece model (some models can break into two pieces, which could be dangerous) with a soft nipple.
- The shield should be made of firm plastic with air holes and be at least 1¼ inches across, so a baby cannot put the entire pacifier into her mouth.

- Make sure the pacifier is dishwasher-safe. Follow the instructions on the pacifier and either boil it or run it through the dishwasher before your baby uses it. Clean it this way frequently until your baby is six months old. After six months, you may clean it by washing it with soap and rinsing it in clear water.
- Pacifiers come in two sizes, one for the first six months and another for children older than six months. For your baby's comfort, make sure the pacifier is the right size.
- There is a variety of nipple shapes. Try different shapes until you find the one your baby prefers.
- Buy some extras. Pacifiers have a way of getting lost or falling on the floor or in the street just when you need them most.
- Never tie a pacifier around your baby's neck or hand, or to your child's crib. This can result in a serious injury or even death
- Do not use the nipple from a baby bottle as a pacifier. If the baby sucks hard, the nipple may pop out of the ring and choke her.
- Pacifiers fall apart over time. Inspect them every once in a while to see whether the rubber has changed colour or has torn. If so, replace them.

Generally, pacifier use in babies does not cause medical or psychological problems. However, pacifiers should generally only be offered when a baby is not hungry: after or between meals. Giving a pacifier to a hungry baby may upset her when she is expecting a meal and not a pacifier.

## Regurgitation and Spitting Up

Spitting up (also known as regurgitation) is something seen very commonly during the first few months. At least 40 percent of normal babies have this problem, which usually occurs immediately after feeding. In adults and older children, there is an elastic-like muscle at the entry to the stomach, which usually closes and prevents liquids from being pushed back up. In babies, however, this band or sphincter is not fully effective, and can easily be pushed back by the contents of the stomach, resulting in spitting up. As you can see, this is not an allergy, a food intolerance, or even vomiting; but rather it is like a bottle with a cap that is not fully closed. If the bottle is filled to the brim with any type of liquid, be it water, milk, or juice, it will overflow through the partially closed cap. If it is moved or tilted, it will also overflow or spill. Understanding this comparison will help you better understand regurgitation and what to do about it.

Logically, it is important not to overload the stomach; therefore, babies who tend to regurgitate should be given less to drink per feed, but more frequently; don't overfeed your baby. In addition, positioning your baby is important. The angle of infant seats can make matters worse and reclining seats should be avoided, especially immediately after a feed. Also, after a feeding, don't move your baby around too vigorously or place her in a position that will cause her to slouch and, therefore, put pressure on her stomach.

Usually, the vast majority of babies outgrow this problem by twelve months or earlier, and their growth and development is not affected at all. A small proportion of babies regurgitate so much that they don't grow properly. For this reason, babies who spit up frequently should be weighed regularly. It's important to be able to tell the difference between vomiting and spitting up, because vomiting may require medical attention. Vomiting is more forceful, and is often accompanied by other symptoms of illness.

# Skin Care and Rashes

## Skin Care and Handling

The skin of a newborn baby is very sensitive, particularly on the face and scalp. Applying lotions or oils to the baby's skin is generally not recommended, because they can clog pores and cause or aggravate rashes. Avoid any products that contain alcohol, artificial colours, preservatives, and other chemical additives, as these can dry or irritate your baby's skin. Also, when bathing, use only baby soaps, which are formulated to be gentle to your baby's sensitive skin. And use non-stinging, non-scented baby shampoo. Be sure to always rinse away soap and shampoo well, using fresh water.

In some normal babies, their skin, especially on the arms and legs, may change colour when being handled, particularly if the surrounding temperature is low. The discoloration looks like a reddish-blue or lacy marbled pattern. This is normal and reflects the immaturity of your baby's blood vessels, which tend to contract or close down abnormally. This subsides over the first six to twelve months of life. Note that if you see blue colour around your baby's mouth or on the lips, it is NOT normal and you should seek medical attention.

## Common Rashes of Newborn Babies

It is very common for babies to have rashes or spots on their skin at birth and during the first few weeks of life. Most of these are not dangerous and go away on their own. Here is a list of some common rashes that we see in newborn babies.

### Erythema Toxicum

Erythema Toxicum is seen in about 50 percent of all full-term babies and can be all over the body except the palms and soles. This rash is much less common in premature babies. Usually, Erythema Toxicum rashes are visible by the second day of life and look like small yellow-white pustules surrounded by a flat red blotchy rash. Your healthcare provider can confirm the rash by examining your baby and may need to take a sample of the pustule for testing to ensure there is no infection. There is no known cause and the rash subsides on its own.

### Hemangioma

Hemangiomas are a type of birthmark that babies are born with or begin to appear within the first few weeks. They are reddish raised bumps that are sometimes referred to as strawberry hemangiomas, because of their look and colour. Appearing on any part of the body, they are thought to be an abnormality of the blood vessels; they usually do not cause any problems and go away without treatment. It is reassuring to know that most hemangiomas typically grow rapidly during the first year and then start to shrink and go away completely by five years of age. Your healthcare provider can give you specific information relevant to your baby.

### Mongolian Spots

Babies can be born with Mongolian spots, which look like flat blotches of faded blue-grey ink. These spots are most commonly on a baby's lower back area and they vary in size. While only 10 percent of Caucasian babies have these spots, they are seen in 80 percent of Black, Asian, and East Indian newborns. There is no known cause or consequence of Mongolian spots; they eventually fade away within the first few years of age.

### Salmon Patch

Salmon patches (also known as nevus simplex) are small patch of skin with a pink discoloration. They are usually seen on the back of the neck, the forehead, and eyelids of newborn babies. Often referred to as stork marks, they are present in about 30 percent to 40 percent of all normal newborn babies. Salmon patches fade away on their own within several months of life and are not dangerous.

### Sebaceous Hyperplasia

These are very tiny yellowish pimples that are frequently seen on a newborn's forehead, nose, cheeks, and upper lips. These are actually sebaceous glands—glands that produce natural oil in the skin—that are swollen at birth and they disappear on their own within the first few weeks.

## Toilet Training

Many parents worry about toilet training their young children. Most of the time, parents will know when their children are ready. However, parents should not rush toilet training nor should they have unrealistic expectations. Patience is key!

Most children are ready to begin toilet training between the ages of two and four, **but certainly not before the age of two**. Remember, each child is different. It takes between three and six months of toilet training before your child is out of diapers for good.

### Signs That a Child Is Ready To Be Toilet Trained

- The child can walk to the potty (or adapted toilet seat).
- The child can sit steadily on the potty.
- The child's diaper remains dry for a few hours in a row.
- The child can follow simple instructions.
- She can let you know when she needs to go.

# Warning Signs of Potentially Serious Problems

## When to Seek Medical Attention

**When a baby is unwell, there are often warning signs. If your baby has any of the following symptoms, seek medical attention right away:**

- Doesn't pass a greenish-black stool within thirty-six hours after birth;
- The skin or the whites of the eyes appear to be turning yellow;
- Stool colour changes to and remains white;
- Vomits forcefully or more frequently than usual;
- Refuses feedings for more than six to eight hours;
- Has a fever before six weeks of age;
- Has a persistent cough;
- Is excessively or uncharacteristically fussy or irritable;
- Is unusually lethargic or sleepy;
- Has colour changes in the lips or face;
- Has bad diarrhea or unusually frequent and very watery stools;
- Appears dehydrated; or
- Has any other unusual symptoms.

**If you're ever worried about your baby's health, never hesitate to seek medical attention.**

# Common Illnesses and Conditions During the First Eighteen Months

As a pediatrician and father, I know that a sick child can be a tremendous source of stress for parents and child caregivers. Often, a lot of this stress is related to the worry of not understanding baby's illness and the feeling of having somehow lost control. By offering useful and practical information, I hope this section will help lessen your anxiety if your child is ill. With a better understanding of your child's condition, you can become better-informed and effective partners with your healthcare provider in managing and safeguarding your baby's health and wellness.

In this section, I have compiled—in alphabetical order—information on childhood illnesses and conditions commonly seen in infants less than eighteen months of age. Note that some of these conditions can be seen in older children, too.

**I would like to stress that the following information may not include each and every affliction of young children and it is not intended to replace the advice of your child's healthcare provider. Rather, this information is offered with the hope that it will complement your present knowledge, any prescribed treatment plans, and consultation with your healthcare provider.**

# Adenoids

Adenoids are tonsil-like glands located at the back of the nose. Although the exact function of adenoids is not understood, it may be related to assisting with protection from infection, but people can live normally without them.

## What Happens to the Adenoids?

Children are born with adenoids that are quite small. As a child grows, so do the adenoids, reaching their maximum size when the child is ten to twelve years old. From that point on, the adenoid tissue starts to shrink on its own. It's during the growth phase that adenoids can potentially cause problems as they get bigger.

## Symptoms of Enlarged Adenoids

Enlarged or hypertrophied adenoids can block a child's nasal passages and result in:

- Nasal congestion;
- Mouth breathing; and/or
- Increased snoring.

In severe cases, where the adenoids block the nasal passage completely, they can cause sleep disturbances. Another clue is a child who is tired all the time as a result of interrupted sleep related to the nasal blockage that typically worsens at night. Very rarely, these complications can be quite dangerous, causing sleep apnea, failure to grow, and even heart failure. Fortunately, however, in the vast majority of children with enlarged adenoids, the main symptoms are just a chronically stuffy nose and/or mouth breathing.

Also, it is important to note that enlarged adenoids are not the only cause of persistent nasal congestion in children.

## Confirming Enlarged Adenoids

Aside from the symptom history, the best way to assess the size of the adenoids is to do a simple X-ray of the neck region, because the adenoids are hidden behind the nose and cannot be seen by direct physical examination. This X-ray reveals two very important details: whether the adenoids are enlarged and, importantly, to what degree they block the nasal passage.

## Treating Enlarged Adenoids

The only treatment for enlarged obstructing adenoids is to surgically remove them. Antibiotics and other medications do not help. The decision to remove the adenoids must come from weighing the benefits of waiting for the adenoids to shrink on their own against the current degree of disruption to a child's life and health. Obviously, in extreme cases, the decision to remove the adenoids is easy to make. In children without extreme symptoms, the decision is usually made on a case-by-case basis, with consultation among the parents, their healthcare provider, and an ENT specialist.

# Allergies and Testing

Up to between 10 percent and 15 percent of all children may have allergic tendencies. Allergy-prone children can either develop asthma, nasal allergies, eczema, and/or food allergies. An allergy develops when a person's body has a bad reaction to a particular substance or product that's normally harmless, such as cow's milk protein or pollens.

The substance that causes the allergic reaction is called an allergen. Allergens can enter the body when they're eaten, touched, or inhaled. They can also enter the body through a bee or wasp sting. (Please see my chapter on Insect Bite Reactions.) When the body perceives the allergen as something harmful, it tries to protect itself by making antibodies to attack the allergen. In the process, the person experiences various allergic symptoms that can range from mild to severe.

## What Are the Allergic Signs?

Many parents of allergic children notice allergic shiners, which are dark circles under her eyes. And worry. However, parents are relieved to find out that shiners are some of the facial features that suggest a child may have allergies; they suggest more specifically that the child is atopic. "Atopic" means that he or she is prone to certain allergic conditions, including nasal allergies, food allergies, hay fever, eczema, and asthma.

Children with these signs are referred to as having allergic facies or atopic facies, and, yes, one sign is the dark circles under the eyes, also known as allergic shiners. Parents often worry that these dark circles under their eyes mean their child is not getting enough sleep. Yet in reality, this is a part of the allergic look and not due to sleep deprivation. Allergic shiners are thought to be caused by increased blood flow near the sinuses.

Another sign we see around the eyes is less obvious. Children with allergies or an atopic tendency tend to have an extra skin fold or line under their lower eyelids. These folds are called Dennie-Morgan lines, named after the doctors who first noticed the relationship between this extra fold of skin and an allergic tendency. Another sign of allergies, more specifically nasal allergies, is the allergic salute. Children with nasal allergies often have an itchy nose, among other symptoms. So as a result, their hand seems always to be scratching their nose as if they are saluting. Frequent throat clearing or hoarseness can be another feature of an allergy as well.

It is important to note that the presence of these signs does not automatically mean the child will develop allergies or related atopic conditions. Indeed, some children may have allergic shiners or an extra lower eyelid skin fold, and have no allergic signs or symptoms at all.

## Are Allergies Inherited?

We know that allergies tend to run in families. More specifically, if one parent has an allergic tendency, then there is about a 40 percent chance that their child will inherit the allergic tendency. If both parents are allergic, then the chance jumps to 75 percent. Even if a child inherits an allergic tendency, he may not necessarily develop allergies during his lifetime. Why some kids who inherit the tendency develop allergies while others don't is not well understood. Also, we do not know why some children show signs of allergies at a very early age, while others only develop their first allergic symptoms well into adulthood.

## Allergy Tests

Allergy testing helps us determine exactly what a person is allergic to by detecting whether a person has developed an antibody against a tested substance such as a specific food, an airborne allergen, or a medication. The easiest and most common way to do this is with the Scratch Test, a simple and relatively painless procedure, in which a series of drops, each containing a specific antigen, is placed on a child's forearm. Next, with a small needle, the area of skin at each drop is pricked very gently. After a ten-minute waiting period, a small bump develops at the site of the scratch when the child has an allergy to the specific substance. The size of the bump and the surrounding redness indicates how much a child is allergic to the specific substance tested.

In general, the test is very safe and does not induce an allergic reaction in the child, other than a local one at the site of the scratch. However, we generally do not perform the test if an asthmatic child has active symptoms at the time of the testing. Allergy tests can be performed at any age. I believe the tests for respiratory allergens give more reliable results in children five years of age and older. We test for food allergies—such as milk protein or peanuts—at any age. Allergy tests can help us identify what specifically is causing an allergic reaction or worsening a child's asthma.

In the case of a food allergy, the test can determine whether a specific food has to be avoided in the diet. In the area of pollen allergies, the situation is more complex. Different pollens appear during different times of the year. Knowing which pollen a child is specifically allergic to can help caregivers better prepare the child during a specific pollen season. Parents often wonder if allergy tests are helpful in determining the cause of eczema in their children. Disappointingly, the answer is usually no.

**It is important to note that** we do not test for cigarette smoke, as everyone is sensitive to the effects of second-hand smoke.

# Apnea

The term "apnea" means no breath, in other words, a stoppage of breathing. In general, this occurs mostly during sleep and is referred to as sleep apnea. In children, there are a number of causes of apnea.

## Central Apnea

In central apnea, the brain's control of breathing is immature or abnormal. The brain controls the muscles we use to breathe. If the brain does not send the signals to the respiratory muscles, breathing stops. If the pause is long enough, this can lead to a decrease in the heart rate, decreased oxygen to the blood, and even death. As a matter of fact, some experts feel that this may be related to SIDS (Sudden Infant Death Syndrome). Similarly, children with brain damage can also have apnea, because the area of the brain that controls breathing may have been damaged or injured.

## Apnea of Prematurity

This is a form of central apnea seen in premature infants who often stop breathing because their brain is too immature to fully control it. As a premature baby gets older, the problem tends to disappear. In the meantime, specific treatments and precautions are usually needed.

## Obstructive Apnea

Obstructive apnea results from a physical blockage of breathing, such as with enlarged adenoids or tonsils. Adenoids and tonsils can get so large that they block the airway, especially during sleep, resulting in breathing pauses or apnea.

## Reflux-Related Apnea

In gastro-esophageal reflux (GE reflux), the acid contents of the stomach are regurgitated back into the esophagus instead of moving downwards toward the intestine. This acidity in the esophagus can sometimes trigger apnea in babies—Reflux-Related Apnea—as a result of the vasovagal reflex.

## What Are the Symptoms of Sleep Apnea?

In some children, the symptoms are obvious: they stop breathing during their sleep. In others, it may be less obvious. For example, they may snore loudly, have periods of on-and-off breathing, or periods of what seem like trying to catch their breath. Many times, children with sleep apnea have disturbed, restless sleep, and wake up tired the next day, because of the frequent nightly apnea episodes.

## What is Periodic Breathing?

Breathing may be irregular in young babies; in other words, the baby may take a few breaths, then pause for a few seconds, then continue again. This is thought to be normal, as they develop and mature their breathing. Apnea, potentially much more serious, is a prolonged stoppage of breathing that can result in low blood oxygen, heart problems, and even death.

## Tests to Confirm Sleep Apnea

The best way to confirm sleep apnea is by doing a sleep study. This test consists of attaching the baby to certain machines that monitor and record his respiratory rate and pattern, oxygen levels, and heart rate. Such tests called sleep studies are performed overnight in a sleep lab. However, some hospitals and medical centres may conduct these studies in the child's home. The sleep study can confirm the presence of sleep apnea, to what degree it is present, and by the pattern of the breathing irregularities can also help distinguish between central or obstructive apnea.

Depending on the individual situation, other tests may be performed, such as certain specific blood tests, a head CAT (computer-assisted tomography, also known as X-ray computed tomography) scan, and an EEG (an electroencephalogram) may be performed to make sure these episodes are not seizures.

In cases where GE reflux is thought to be the cause, a pH study to determine the level of acidity in the esophagus may be performed as well, preferably at the same time as the sleep study. In this way, the specialist reviewing the overnight study can relate the apnea to the reflux; in other words, the apnea occurs whenever the pH of the esophagus becomes acidic due to the contents of the stomach re-entering the esophagus.

## How Is Apnea Treated?

### Obstructive Apnea

Apnea treatment depends on its cause. If a child has obstructive apnea, then the adenoids and/or tonsils are removed and this generally cures the condition. In older individuals, a night-time respirator machine may be needed. Called a CPAP (continuous positive airway pressure) machine, this is attached to a mask worn during sleep. The machine gently pushes air into the airways constantly to ensure that there is no pause in respiration. (This is rarely required in children and is most common in adults.)

### GE Reflux Apnea

If the cause is due to GE reflux, then the reflux is treated and the apnea improves as well.

### Central Apnea

There really is no specific treatment for central apnea. In this case, depending on the situation, the baby may be put on a home apnea monitor that rings whenever she has an episode. In this case, parents are trained to perform CPR (cardiopulmonary resuscitation) and are followed and supported by a specialized sleep apnea team. If and when the apnea resolves or improves depends on the individual situation.

### Apnea of Prematurity

Apnea of prematurity is sometimes treated with caffeine or similar products. These treatments are thought to work by stimulating the premature baby's respiratory control centre. As the baby gets older, the apnea usually resolves.

# Asthma

Asthma (also known as reactive airway disease) can affect up to 10 percent of children and most commonly starts within the first two years of life. In most case, it decreases or goes away completely by the age of eight.

## Symptoms of Asthma

There are two main problems associated with asthma: bronchoconstriction and inflammation. Bronchoconstriction means that the airways or bronchi close down or constrict. Inflammation means that the airways are irritated and full of secretions. Both of these problems block the bronchi and cause the typical asthma symptoms, which include shortness of breath, wheezing, and/or coughing. Sometimes these symptoms occur alone, sometimes in different combinations. Other respiratory illnesses have similar symptoms. But in children with asthma, these symptoms usually keep coming back, so it's important to also recognize a pattern or history of symptoms.

The most common symptom is wheezing, which is a high-pitched breathing sound, especially noticeable as the child breathes out. Other indicators of a more serious episode include rapid breathing, prolonged exhaling, or an exaggerated use (tugging or pulling) of the muscles in the chest and neck to assist breathing. It's important that parents and caregivers are able to recognize asthma symptoms, to help determine its severity and the need for medication, and to help monitor the effectiveness of the child's treatment program.

Still, a child can have asthma even though he never wheezes. In fact, about 5 percent of asthmatic children have a cough as their only symptom. It's also possible that a child who has frequent or prolonged cold symptoms actually has asthma, even though they've yet to have a recognizable asthma attack.

## Making the Diagnosis

Before discussing the actual asthma test, it is important to know that most children who develop asthma do so in the first few years of life. The diagnosis is made by the history of symptoms. It is generally agreed that if a child has repetitive episodes of shortness of breath and/or wheezing and/or a cough and has no other lung problems, the diagnosis of asthma can be made.

For those children younger than six years of age, the diagnosis of asthma is usually based on a history of symptoms. In older children, special breathing tests can help in the assessment of asthma. But because most children develop asthma within the first two years of life, a history of symptoms is often all we have to rely on.

Children often develop a pattern of symptoms that parents can learn to recognize. Recognizing these patterns can help you and your healthcare provider determine effective treatment. Remember, however, that asthma symptoms change and new ones can appear in the same child. As time goes by, you'll be able to recognize the signs of an oncoming attack earlier!

## How Is Asthma Affected by the Environment?

Asthma is most often triggered in children by a respiratory infection, such as the common cold. But the presence of other irritants—especially cigarette smoke; tiny insects called dust mites; animal dander, especially from cats; plant pollen; air pollution; deodorants and perfumes—often make asthma symptoms more frequent, more severe, and more difficult to control. Other asthma triggers that can bring on an immediate asthma attack include, exercise, cold air, and—in older children—emotional stress.

Asthma symptoms often appear immediately after exposure to a trigger. But sometimes the presence of such things as dust or cigarette smoke can have less obvious immediate effects—though still be harmful. Sometimes symptoms appear only hours or even days after exposure. This can make it difficult to identify what a child reacted to. For example, a child may play with a cat and seem to have no immediate symptoms. But in a so-called late reaction, symptoms appear only later on, which is the result of inflammation.

Inflammation resulting from irritants can increase the child's sensitivity to such triggers as those mentioned above. In other words, a child constantly exposed to irritants such as cigarette smoke or dust mites is more susceptible to having an asthma attack brought on by a trigger—such as a cold—as compared to a child not regularly exposed to irritants.

By decreasing your child's exposure to environmental irritants and allergens, you can actually reduce your child's need for medication. Maintaining a healthy breathing environment is an essential part of the treatment program.

## Asthma Tests

Testing for asthma is not that simple. The only test that can prove the child has asthma is the provocation test, in which children breathe in a substance known to close down the bronchi or airway tubes. Ordinarily, at a certain dose, everyone will react to this medication (histamine or methacoline) and their bronchi will close down or constrict, which can be measured by the rate at which one breathes out.

Peak Flow Meters are devices that can be used at home to assess a child's asthma. These tests, only possible in school-age or older children, determine how quickly a child can breathe out—a measure of airway blockage at that time—and are used to monitor a child's symptoms on a daily basis. A normal test in this instance neither confirms nor eliminates the diagnosis of asthma.

Given that asthma testing is not possible in the majority of asthmatics who are younger than school age, the diagnosis, follow-up treatment, and decisions to modify treatment are based solely on the symptoms. This is why I always recommend keeping a daily asthma diary, which is the best way to document a child's asthmatic symptoms and progress. Parents should record the following: the presence of day or night-time symptoms, dates of hospitalizations or emergency room visits, and, very importantly, the need for bronchodilator use. This last measurement is a very good indication of the degree of asthma control. Asthmatic children requiring less than five bronchodilator doses per week are usually considered to have the condition well controlled.

## Treating Asthma

Once diagnosed with asthma, your child will probably be prescribed specific medication. Just as there are two main problems associated with asthma—bronchoconstriction and inflammation—there are two main types of asthma medications: bronchodilators and anti-inflammatory drugs.

Asthma inhalers—also known as puffers and medication delivery systems—have been designed to deliver medication directly to the lungs. This results both in quicker and more efficient action and less medication entering into the bloodstream. Prior to the development of inhalers, the medications used to treat asthma and other respiratory conditions were taken by mouth in pill or liquid form. Medication taken by mouth is swallowed into the stomach and ultimately enters the bloodstream to then travel to the target area—the bronchi (airway tubes). This indirect route is less effective than the inhaled route. Also, because oral asthmatic medications enter the bloodstream, there is, of course, the potential for more side effects. Asthma inhalers allow medication to go directly into the airways, thus maximizing effectiveness yet with potentially fewer side effects.

## Are There Different Types of Inhalers?

Yes, there are two main categories of puffers:

1. Aerosol or spray puffers are called Metered Dose Inhalers (MDIs). MDIs eject medication in an aerosol form into the lungs. The medication is mixed with a gas to make it spray easily. This gas used to be CFC (chlorofluorocarbon), but for environmental reasons, MDIs today are CFC-free. Children must be at least eight to nine years old to able to use these devices properly, as they require quite a bit of coordination. With the end of the puffer in the mouth, the child has to breathe in while pressing down on the inhaler to release the spray. In order to allow the administration of puffers to younger children, devices called spacers have been developed. Basically, spacers are tubes into which the MDI puffer fits on one end. The other end of the spacer is either a mouthpiece for children older than five years of age or a mask for younger children and infants. Various types of medication can be found in MDI puffers—bronchodilator medications that open up the airway or corticosteroid medications that prevent asthma attacks. Some puffers contain combinations of two medications.
2. The other category of asthma medication delivery systems is the dry powder system. These devices, used by children over five years of age, contain medication in powder form. The devices are placed into the mouth and the child breathes in the medication by sucking in, just like sucking on a straw. As with the MDI puffers, the medications in the devices are either a bronchodilator, a cortisone, or both.

In certain situations, children are prescribed cortisone-containing devices on a daily, preventative basis, and the bronchodilator puffer is to be used as needed, rather than regularly. I know this all sounds confusing, but when parents understand how to use the prescribed puffers properly, their child's asthma can usually be controlled very well. Which inhaler and which type of medication is prescribed depend on the age and individual situation of the child.

The main point is that inhalers have played a big role in our ability to improve asthma control in children. Used properly and appropriately, asthma delivery devices are safe and extremely effective!

# Bed Bugs

Recently there have been many media reports about bed bugs. Authorities have now recognized them as a growing problem and are implementing public awareness and prevention campaigns. It is important to note that there are no known cases of infectious diseases transmitted by bed bugs. However, scratching a bitten area may lead to infection. Nevertheless, bed bugs can certainly be a nuisance and an inconvenience and, in large numbers, may cause their victims great discomfort.

## About Bed Bugs

Bed bugs, also known as *Cimex lectularius*, are tiny, wingless insects. Active mostly at night, they are very small (about the size of an apple seed), oval, and rusty red in colour. After feeding on human blood, they become bigger and easier to see. They are often hiding in places like cracks in furniture, floors, and walls, behind headboards, in mattress seams, along baseboard cracks, and in other bedroom items, including window and door casings, pictures, mouldings, cracks in plaster, and loose wallpaper.

In North America, cases of bed bugs were rampant before World War II. Post-war, thanks to collective efforts and new pest-control techniques, they ceased to exist. However, their reappearance is thought to be a result of the bugs being inadvertently carried into North America from other countries.

## How Do Bed Bugs Get Into Homes?

Bed bugs get carried into people's homes without them knowing it, in items such as luggage or clothing. They can be picked up in high-traffic areas like hotels, boarding houses, airplanes, ships, and buses. Be aware that second-hand furniture including mattresses may also carry bed bugs into your home.

## Signs That Your Home Has Bed Bugs

- Large, itchy rashes on skin;
- Small linen or mattress bloodstains (from crushed bugs);
- Seeing the bed bugs themselves.

## How To Handle Bed Bug Bites

If you have been bitten by a bed bug, clean your skin, and keep it clean to prevent infection. Try not to scratch the bite. If it is itchy, antihistamine (an anti-allergy medication) may be recommended by your healthcare provider or pharmacist.

## Getting Rid of Bed Bugs

Here are some important steps that are helpful in getting rid of bed bugs:

- Using a stiff brush, remove bed bugs (and their eggs) from mattress seams.
- Vacuum sleeping areas frequently. Pay special attention to carpets, mattresses, bed frames, furniture, wall cracks, and floor cracks. After vacuuming, seal the vacuum bag in a plastic bag and dispose of it in an outdoor container.
- Steam-clean all carpets (not mattresses).
- Repair loose wallpaper and cracked plaster and fill any other cracks in your home.
- Place infested items in a tightly sealed plastic bag place in an outdoor container.
- Do not resell or donate infested furniture or clothing.

- Note that sometimes it is difficult get rid of bed bugs on your own; you may need to hire a licensed pest-control specialist.

## Preventing Bed Bugs From Entering Your Home

The best way to prevent bed bugs in your home is to:

- Wash and inspect clothing and luggage immediately after every trip; and
- Never bring discarded furniture into your home. Buyer beware at second-hand furniture sales!

# Breath-Holding Spells

Breath-holding spells are episodes during intense crying when a child will seemingly stop breathing, become pale or even blue, and go limp. Prolonged or intense crying leads to the involuntary holding of breath resulting in the child appearing to stop breathing. Although this is quite scary for parents, fortunately, there are no serious consequences.

## What Is the Cause of Breath-Holding Spells?

It is not known why certain children have breath-holding spells, but it is known that they are all preceded by an intense period of crying, usually out of frustration. They occur equally frequently in males and females. There is a family history of breath-holding spells in about 25 percent of cases. These episodes are not seizures, nor do they cause a lack of oxygen to the brain.

## What Can Parents Do?

The first thing is not to panic. Here are some other helpful tips:

- Quickly apply a cold cloth to the face or gently tap the child's cheeks. If this is done in the first fifteen seconds of the breath-holding, this may end the spell.
- Put the child on the floor or in the crib to prevent injury from falling during unconsciousness.
- Do not lift the child vertically upwards; this may actually make things worse. When picking up the child do so while the child is lying horizontally.

Discuss this situation with your healthcare provider. Although in most cases the diagnosis is simple to make, sometimes the healthcare provider may perform specific tests to make sure that the spells are not seizures or the result of epilepsy. In most situations, the child is well otherwise, and the pattern of the spells and the fact that crying sets them off is enough to confirm the diagnosis of breath-holding spells.

## Will Children Outgrow Breath-Holding Spells?

Yes. Breath-holding spells usually begin after six months of age and peak at about age two. Most children outgrow breath-holding spells by the age of five years.

Also, more rarely in young children, breath-holding spells can be brought on by a painful injury such as a fall on the head or a severe fright, without intense crying. This is similar to adult fainting spells due to the so-called vasovagal reflex that causes the heart to slow resulting in paleness, limpness, and even loss of consciousness. Interestingly, many adults who suffer from easy fainting when seeing blood or with a minor injury had breath-holding spells as young children.

## Can Breath-Holding Spells Be Prevented?

Breath-holding spells are usually due to a child being frustrated. So, trying to limit, foresee, or even prevent frustrating experiences may prevent an episode. Also avoid situations like fatigue and hunger, which always make things worse. Setting firm consistent limits will also help a child deal better with frustration.

# Bronchiolitis

Every year, many babies develop bronchiolitis and some develop it so badly that they have to be admitted to hospital. Bronchiolitis is an infection of the bronchioles, the small airways (tubes) within the lungs.

## What Causes Bronchiolitis?

The Respiratory Syncytial Virus—known commonly as RSV—causes the bronchiolitis infection, which usually develops during the winter or early spring. RSV usually causes the typical bronchiolitis symptoms described below in children less than two years of age. In older people, it usually causes infections that resemble the common cold.

The typical symptoms of bronchiolitis in babies include:

- Cough;
- Wheezing;
- Difficulty breathing;
- Production of large amounts of secretions; and
- Decreased feeding or drinking.

**If your baby has any of the above symptoms, you should seek medical attention immediately.**

## Bronchiolitis Treatment

Because bronchiolitis is caused by a virus, antibiotics are not effective in treating RSV. An antiviral medication (Ribavirin) has been tested. Because of its potential side effects and impracticality of use, this medication is not generally used. Therefore, the treatment is supportive and depends on the severity of the infection. Most infants with RSV bronchiolitis cough and/or wheeze a bit, but in general, they feed well and do not need oxygen or any other treatment. Within a few days their infection clears on its own.

## More Severe Cases of Bronchiolitis

Some babies may have enough discomfort and difficulty from the wheezing and secretions that they may need extra oxygen, or even the administration of Ventolin or salbutamol (a bronchodilator used in asthma). Also, if they cannot drink enough, they may require an intravenous. One of the most important aspects of treatment is helping these babies get rid of their excessive secretions and this usually requires hospitalization. Rarely, in very severe cases, some babies are actually placed on respirators to help them breathe.

### Are Any Babies at High Risk?

Premature babies and those with chronic respiratory or cardiac problems are at higher risk for developing severe bronchiolitis. Because of this, a special vaccine has been developed for these high-risk babies that offers protection against RSV. If you have a baby who is at high risk for RSV, you should speak to your healthcare provider.

### Is Bronchiolitis Asthma?

The issue about RSV becoming asthma is potentially confusing, because the symptoms of bronchiolitis are the same as those of asthma. Asthma is defined as a condition of recurrent episodes of wheezing and/or coughing and/or difficulty breathing in a child with no other lung problems or conditions. There is some uncertainty as to the relationship of RSV infection and the subsequent development of asthma. Some experts suggest that children who have an inherited allergic or asthmatic tendency are more prone to RSV infections, while others say that RSV may trigger subsequent asthma. In any case, if a child seems to be getting recurrent episodes of coughing and breathing difficulties, asthma would be the more likely cause rather than recurrent bronchiolitis. However, if a child has had only one isolated RSV episode and nothing else later on, then by definition, this is not asthma.

# Chickenpox

Chickenpox (also known as varicella) is a very contagious easy-to-spread infection caused by the varicella-zoster virus. Chickenpox is a very common childhood infection. Most children by the age of nine will have had chickenpox.

This virus is spread from one person to another in one of two ways:

- By direct contact with the actual rash; or
- Through the  air by coughing or sneezing, just like with a cold.

## Chickenpox Symptoms

The symptoms of chickenpox vary from child to child. Some children develop such a mild form of chickenpox that their parents do not even realize that they have had it. However, in typical cases, the disease starts with one or more of the following symptoms:

- Fever;
- Cold-like symptoms;
- Fatigue;
- Irritability.

Within a day or so, the typical chickenpox rash develops, which is a very characteristic one and usually easy to identify. The rash begins as a round or oval red spot that develops a blister-like centre full of a yellowish fluid containing the varicella virus. The rash, which can be quite itchy, may occur anywhere on the body. Some children develop very few blisters while others seem to have their whole body covered.

## When Is Chickenpox Contagious?

A child developing chickenpox is considered to be contagious a couple of days before the rash actually breaks out. This is why the disease spreads so easily, as children are contagious before the rash comes out and generally are still attending school or daycare. Once the rash appears, the child is contagious for about three to five days, or until all the blisters have dried and crusted off. Only when all the lesions are crusted can a child return to school or daycare.

### Incubation Period

Parents often wonder how long it takes to develop the illness after being exposed to a child with chickenpox. This period—known as the incubation period—ranges between eleven and twenty days, although for most children it develops within fourteen days. If a child does not develop chickenpox after this period, then he or she has not been infected this time.

## What Are the Complications of Chickenpox?

Fortunately, most children do not suffer any serious consequences from chickenpox infections. From a cost-to-society point of view, chickenpox can be expensive and inconvenient. Because children have to miss school, parents have to miss work, causing inconvenience and a loss of productivity all around. However, approximately one in two thousand children may develop more serious complications, requiring hospitalization. These complications include:

- Pneumonia;
- Bacterial infection of the rash, and, rarely, flesh-eating disease;
- Brain inflammation or encephalitis;

- Balance problems related to infection of a specific part of the brain (cerebellitis); and
- Death (very rare).

### Who Is Particularly Susceptible to Chickenpox?

Varicella zoster infections are more serious or dangerous in the following groups of high-risk individuals):

- Adults;
- Very young children;
- Adults or children with weak immune systems (such as those with AIDS or cancer);
- People on medications that weaken their immune systems (such as oral cortisone).

## What Is the Treatment for Chickenpox?

There is no specific recommended treatment or medicine for healthy children who develop chickenpox. The general approach to uncomplicated chickenpox infections includes the following:

- Applications of calamine lotion;
- Soothing baths of oatmeal, baking soda, or cornstarch to help relieve the itch;
- Cool compresses may also help;
- Making sure children have short nails so they don't scratch and infect the rash; young babies may need mittens;
- For temperature control, acetaminophen can be given as needed for age and weight;
- **ASA or aspirin should never be given to children with chickenpox.** When given with certain viral infections including

chickenpox and influenza, ASA has been associated with a sometimes fatal condition called Reye's syndrome that can result in liver and brain damage.
- Make sure they are drinking well (and enough);
- If a child is having difficulty eating because of chickenpox in the mouth, offer him cold fluids (avoid acid drinks like apple or orange juice) and a soft diet.

For high-risk individuals who either develop or are exposed to varicella infection, there are certain antiviral medications and other treatments that may need to be given to protect their weakened bodies. In many cases, they will require hospitalization.

### When to Seek Medical Attention?

You should see a healthcare provider if:

- Signs of infection such as redness or swelling develop around the blisters;
- There is a very high fever;
- The child vomits more than three times;
- The child is confused, difficult to awaken, or has trouble walking;
- You are worried that your child is not following the typical course of chickenpox (as compared with another child).

### Can Chickenpox Be Prevented by a Vaccine?

Yes, there is a vaccine that protects children from chickenpox. The vaccine has been proven to be 85 percent effective in preventing the disease and almost 100 percent effective in preventing severe disease. Obviously, this results in a decrease of potential complications.

## About Shingles

Chicken pox and shingles (also known as Zoster or Zona) are actually caused by the same virus. However, there are differences in the way the infection develops and spreads. Also, the chicken pox form of the infection is far more common in children than is the shingles form.

It is known that after a chickenpox infection, the varicella virus remains in our bodies forever. The virus remains "asleep" in our nerves. For a variety of reasons, usually in older people or those with weakened immune systems, the virus appears on the skin again. However, this time it only comes out in an area fed by one or more nerves, called a dermatome. It looks like a localized "patch of varicella blisters." This is called Herpes Zoster or shingles.

While we usually see shingles in the elderly, or individuals with weakened immune systems, it can occur in otherwise normal children too, but much less frequently.

People who have not yet had chicken pox or the varicella vaccination can actually contract the virus and develop typical chicken pox infection from someone who has shingles. More specifically, if they come into contact with the little blisters that actually contain the varicella zoster virus. A person with zoster is considered contagious until the blisters (vesicles) have dried and crusted. Persons who have had chicken pox in the past or have been vaccinated will be protected, whether they come into contact with active typical chickenpox or shingles.

# Colds and Coughs

There are several hundred viruses that cause the common cold. The symptoms include runny or stuffy nose, mild cough, and low-grade fever. The common cold is spread through respiratory droplets directly from sneezing and coughing. These viruses can also be spread indirectly by touching an infected surface and then placing your hand close to your face without first washing it. Colds usually go away on their own within a few days. Most babies and toddlers with colds may be less hungry, but still manage to drink well and recover fully.

## Treating Colds and Coughs

There is no specific treatment as colds go away on their own. However, parents often ask about over-the-counter (OTC) cold and cough syrups or preparations, especially if their child is uncomfortable or cannot sleep. It is important to note that OTC **cold and cough preparations are not recommended for children under six years of age**. In fact, studies have shown them to be ineffective for this age group and to have potentially serious side effects.

The basic treatment of a cold includes a humidifier (I prefer cold air mists), drinking plenty of fluids, and for younger children, helping wash out the congested nose with a nose pump and saline (salt-water) drops. In most situations, these simple techniques combined with Tender Loving Care (TLC) do the trick.

# Conjunctivitis

Conjunctivitis (also known as pinkeye) is an irritation or inflammation of the conjunctiva, the covering that lines the inside of the eyelids and the whites of the eyes.

## What Causes Conjunctivitis?

There are three major causes of conjunctivitis:

- Infectious conjunctivitis: (probably the most common). This is caused by a bacterial or viral infection.
- Allergic conjunctivitis: This is due to airborne pollen or dust or something similar getting into the eye.
- Chemical conjunctivitis : Many types of chemicals like sprays, perfumes, deodorants, and household cleaners can irritate the conjunctiva.

## Symptoms of Conjunctivitis

- Red or pink eyes;
- Itchiness or irritation (feeling like sand is in the eye);
- Watery eyes;
- Eye pain;
- A thick, sticky, yellowish discharge. In viral conjunctivitis, the discharge is usually clear.

## Is Infectious Conjunctivitis Contagious?

**Yes.** Many types of bacteria and viruses can cause conjunctivitis in children. These germs can pass from person to person through contact with infected body fluids such as eye discharge; they can also spread on a child's hands if he rubs or wipes his infected eyes. It is important that children not share towels or washcloths, and that they wash before and after meals and touching their faces. The same goes for parents and caretakers after they have contacted the facial or eye area of a child with infectious conjunctivitis.

## How Is Conjunctivitis Treated?

The treatment depends on the cause.

**Bacterial conjunctivitis** is treated with antibiotics, either eye drops or an ointment. With certain types of bacteria, oral antibiotics may be needed. Gentle eye compresses using a clean cotton ball or washcloths soaked in warm water may help, especially before applying any prescribed antibiotic drops or ointments. Ask your healthcare provider when your child can return to school.

**Viral conjunctivitis** cannot be treated with antibiotics effectively, but it usually clears up on its own after a few days. Viral conjunctivitis is also contagious, so follow your healthcare provider's advice about when your child can return to school. Warm compresses may help too.

**Allergic conjunctivitis** is usually treated with oral antihistamines and decongestants or with antihistamine eye drops. Cool compresses may also help.

## When to Seek Medical Attention

Call your healthcare provider if your child has any of the following symptoms:

- Unusually red, itchy, or watery eyes;
- Puffy or swollen eyes;
- Thick, sticky, yellowish discharge coming from the eyes;

- Eyelids that look crusty or stick together when your child awakens;
- Your child complains that his vision is not normal;
- The area under the lower eyelid is red or swollen.

# Cow's Milk Protein Allergy

Cow's milk allergy is the most common food allergy in young children. Fortunately, most babies outgrow milk allergies by their second or third year. In the meantime, parents of babies with milk allergies can be reassured that—although there is no treatment that can cure milk allergies—symptoms can be controlled through a dairy-free diet.

## What Is Cow's Milk (Protein) Allergy?

Regular cow's milk is made up of protein, carbohydrates (sugars), fat, vitamins, minerals, and water. It's the milk protein that causes the allergic reaction in cow's milk allergy. Cow's milk protein allergy can develop in both breastfed and formula-fed children. However, breastfed children are usually less likely to develop food allergies of any sort. Occasionally, though, breastfed children develop cow's milk allergy when they react to the slight amount of cow's milk protein that passes from their mother's diet into her breast milk. In other cases, certain babies can become sensitized to the cow's milk protein in their mother's breast milk, but don't actually have an allergic reaction until they're later introduced to cow's milk themselves.

## Symptoms of Cow's Milk Protein Allergy

Babies who develop cow's milk protein allergy may have one or several of the following symptoms:

- Eczema or skin rash;
- Abdominal pain or cramps;
- Vomiting;
- Diarrhea.

Less commonly, some children may have a very serious allergic reaction called anaphylaxis. This reaction usually occurs within minutes after eating or drinking food to which they're allergic. The most serious symptom of an anaphylactic reaction is the swelling of the face, mouth, and tongue leading to difficulty breathing. Hives, itchy rash, flushing, and severe vomiting are other signs that may be present should an anaphylactic reaction occur. If your child ever has these symptoms, get medical help immediately, because untreated anaphylaxis can quickly become fatal. Fortunately, anaphylaxis is rare.

## How Is Cow's Milk Allergy Confirmed?

There are two very important reasons for making sure that a healthcare provider evaluates your baby's condition to confirm whether or not she has a milk allergy. The first reason is that cow's milk allergy is not the only cause of abdominal pain, eczema, rash, vomiting, diarrhea, or excessive crying. These symptoms can be caused by other conditions, which would need a different treatment. The second reason is because of the danger of an anaphylactic reaction. It's extremely important to know for certain if your child has a cow's milk protein allergy, because if she does, you'll have to be very careful about making sure that all milk and milk products are removed from her diet.

Because each child is unique, a baby with a suspected milk allergy should have an individualized medical assessment, treatment plan, and follow up. After the healthcare provider has carefully reviewed your child's medical history, he or she may recommend that you modify your diet if you're breastfeeding, or that you switch formulas. The healthcare provider may recommend, in some mild cases, reintroducing milk after a month or so on a dairy-free diet, to see whether the child still has symptoms of milk allergy. In other cases, the healthcare provider may refer the child to an allergist. The allergist will try to determine the cause of the baby's symptoms, by doing a skin test or by taking a special blood test.

## How Is Cow's Milk Allergy Treated?

### The Breastfed Child

If you're breastfeeding, and your child has been diagnosed with a cow's milk allergy, you don't need to stop breastfeeding. In fact, your baby's allergic symptoms can be relieved by simply removing dairy products from your own diet, as well as from your baby's. Your healthcare provider can advise you about a healthy, dairy-free diet that would be appropriate for you.

### The Formula-Fed Child

Unlike lactose intolerance, cow's milk protein allergy can be very dangerous. A child with cow's milk allergy should not be given any dairy products at all. Babies on formula who have cow's milk allergy are given special formulas containing no cow's milk protein. They are usually soy-based products (Isomil®, ProSobee®, and Nursoy®) or hydrolysate formulas (Nutramigen® and Alimentum®). In this case, switching from one type of regular infant formula to another is not an option, because all regular formulas contain cow's milk protein. Additionally, lactose-free cow's milk or formulas should not be given to cow's milk allergic children, because they need to completely avoid cow's milk protein.

If the child has been diagnosed with a severe milk allergy, the healthcare provider may prescribe special medications in addition to a dairy-free diet. These medications, such as antihistamines or epinephrine (EpiPen® or AllerjetTM ), are to be used as directed if your child accidentally consumes dairy products and experiences an allergic reaction.

### When Can Baby Restart Dairy Products?

Most children will outgrow their milk allergy within the first two years of life, but they should have an allergy test before restarting diets containing cow's milk protein. Each case varies and this is why it is important to discuss these specifics with your child's healthcare provider. Your healthcare provider will probably recommend that your child's diet be free of dairy products for at least the first twelve to eighteen months. He or she may then retest the child every six months until she determines that your baby is no longer allergic to cow's milk. Once your healthcare provider confirms that your child has outgrown the milk allergy, make sure to follow her recommendations as to how to introduce dairy foods back into the diet. But until your healthcare provider tells you that it is safe to do so, don't try to reintroduce milk into your child's diet on your own.

And if milk or milk products have ever caused an immediate, severe reaction—or anaphylaxis—you should never under any circumstances reintroduce it into your child's diet unless allergy tests have confirmed that your child has outgrown the allergy. In those severe cases, it may sometimes be recommended to introduce milk into your child's diet under close medical supervision, such as in a hospital setting.

## What Other Foods or Products Need To Be Avoided?

When your baby starts eating solid foods, you'll have to be very careful not to give her cow's milk or any food containing milk or milk products for as long as she remains allergic to milk. And if you have any doubts about what's in a particular food, it's best to play it safe and not give it to your child.

Here's a helpful list of some foods and food ingredients to avoid:

- Any type of cow's milk or food containing cow's milk (including skim, dried, solid, evaporated, and condensed).
- Lactaid®, which is milk that has been specially processed for lactose intolerant people. Lactaid® still contains cow's milk protein, and so should not be given to children with milk allergy.

- Cheese, cheese curds, yogurt, and ice cream.
- Butter and buttermilk. Also, many margarines have milk in them, so be sure to carefully check the ingredients.
- Soy products containing cow's milk. Many of the popular soy-based products now on the market, such as frozen soy desserts, actually contain small amounts of cow's milk. So, again, be sure to read labels carefully for product ingredients.
- Pre-mixed cereals containing powdered cow's milk.
- Any products containing casein, caseinate (either sodium caseinate or calcium caseinate), lactalbumin, and whey. These terms all indicate the presence of milk protein.

This list only shows you some of the foods to avoid, so be sure to consult your healthcare provider for more information about which other foods should be removed from your child's diet.

## Can a Cow's Milk Protein Allergic Child Eat Beef?

Parents often wonder whether their child with cow's milk protein allergy can eat beef, since milk and beef both come from cows. Recent studies show that such children only rarely have problems eating beef or veal. Therefore, most milk allergic children can eat beef without any problem.

## What Can Parents Tell Their Allergic Child?

As your child gets older, explain his condition to him in understandable terms. Teach him to never accept food from friends or other people, and about how to be cautious without being fearful. Also, be creative in your preparation of meals, so that they still look and taste good even though they're dairy-free. Your child will feel more comfortable with a diet if it's similar to what those around him are eating.

# Croup

Croup is caused by an inflammation (swelling) of the upper airway, the larynx and the trachea (also known as the voice box and the windpipe). The inflammation is usually due to a viral infection, and is a common condition in young children. Croup is also known as stridorous laryngitis. Viral croup is more common in children less than five years of age and is very rarely seen in adults.

## Symptoms of Croup

Typically, viral croup begins with a cold that slowly develops into a characteristic seal-like barking cough and a high-pitched, raspy noise when breathing in, known as stridor. The stridor often gets worse with physical activity. Most children with viral croup have a low-grade fever. The potential problems of croup depend on how much the upper airway is blocked by the swelling. The more the airway is blocked, the more the child's breathing is laboured and in general the less the child is active. Additionally, an important sign of difficulty in breathing is that the child may stop eating and drinking. Croup typically worsens at night, lasts for three to four days, and usually subsides on its own. Often the severity of the croup is measured by the Croup Score, which takes into account a child's breathing rate and pattern, and the colour of the child's face and lips. The higher the score, the more severe the infection. The croup scores help medical personnel classify the croup as mild, moderate, or severe.

## How Is Croup Treated?

The cough and stridor of croup may be quite scary, but fortunately, most cases are mild and need no treatment or medical intervention. The type of treatment (if any) depends on the severity of the symptoms.

The treatment approach is simple: exposure to cold humid air. This is achieved by either opening up a window or taking the child outside. Another way is to let the shower run, preferably with cold water, and to let the child sit in the bathroom to breathe in the cold humid mist. Usually, children start to breathe more easily within fifteen minutes of exposure to cold humid air. During the rest of the croup illness, a cold-water humidifier or vaporizer in the room during the night is also recommended.

## Moderate to Severe Croup

In the most serious cases, a child may have so much difficulty breathing that she is not getting enough oxygen into the blood. In this situation, the child will need to go to the hospital. Signs that a child with croup needs immediate medical attention include:

- Stridor that is getting louder with each breath;
- Inability to speak because of lack of breath;
- Laboured and or rapid breathing;
- Pale or bluish mouth or fingernails;
- Stridor at rest;
- Drooling;
- Inability to eat or drink enough.

At the hospital, the child will be evaluated and given oxygen if necessary. In order to ensure that the child does not become dehydrated, an intravenous may be started. Although there are no specific medications for croup, steroid injections and adrenaline-like inhaled preparations are used to help children with moderate to severe croup. These medications act to decrease the swelling of the upper airway.

## Can Croup Recur?

Yes. Some children seem to have repeated episodes of croup, called spasmodic croup. In this case, the child gets a cold, rarely with fever, and then the typical croup begins. In some cases, spasmodic croup may begin suddenly without any preceding cold symptoms. Unlike viral croup, spasmodic croup usually recurs, can occur in older children, and is thought to be related to allergies. Of course, in rare cases if a child suffers from repeated episodes of severe croup requiring hospitalization, specific tests are performed by an ENT specialist to ensure there are no vocal cord or other laryngeal problems or anomalies. Fortunately, in the vast majority of children with viral and/or spasmodic croup, there is no underlying airway abnormality.

## Daycare Infections

Many parents are shocked to discover their young children tend to get a lot of infections (up to twelve to fourteen per year) when first attending daycare, because they are constantly exposed to germs from one another. As they get older, this number decreases.

How can you prevent infections? First of all, immunization is very important. Proper nutrition is of course another vital element. Whether or not vitamins help prevent infections in a child who eats a well-balanced diet is an area that is not clear. Breastfeeding is by far the very best nutrition both from the dietary and from the infection-prevention points of view. Mother's antibodies passed to baby in the breast milk will help protect him against infections including the common daycare-associated infections, such as gastroenteritis and ear infections.

**The best thing that the daycare can do is practise infection-control techniques, especially washing hands before and after every child contact.**

# Ear Infections

An ear infection (also known as otitis media) occurs when an infection develops behind the eardrum, in the area known as the middle ear. Normally, the middle ear is filled with air, allowing the eardrum to vibrate and, therefore, transmit sounds to the brain. But sometimes when a person has a cold or other respiratory illness, the middle ear fills with fluid. In adults, this fluid usually drains naturally through the Eustachian tube, which extends downward from the middle ear to the back of the nose. But in young children, the Eustachian tube often drains poorly, because the tube isn't mature or strong enough, and because it extends horizontally rather than downward. As a result, fluid can build up in the middle ear. Bacteria from the nasal passages can easily invade this fluid and cause an ear infection. This is why otitis media occurs so often during or shortly after a cold, when the nose is congested or stuffy.

## Symptoms of an Ear Infection

- Earache;
- Irritability, increased crying, and fussiness;
- Fever; and
- Discharge from the ear.
- Infants who cannot yet speak may tug at or rub their ears.

## The Ear Infection Prone Child

There are a number of factors that may contribute to a tendency toward a child having repeated ear infections.

- A history of ear infections in the family;
- Regular exposure to tobacco smoke;

- A history of allergies;
- Exposure to many other children such as in a daycare setting;
- A history of having been bottle-fed, rather than breastfed during infancy;
- Putting the baby to bed with a bottle or a pacifier;
- Facial deformities associated with cleft palate or Down's syndrome;
- Onset of a first ear infection before six months of age.

## How Middle Ear Infections Are Treated

Otitis media is usually treated with antibiotics that are taken by mouth, prescribed for a total of five to ten days, depending on the antibiotic selected. Symptoms should start to improve within forty-eight hours after starting the antibiotics. In the meantime, if needed, acetaminophen may be given for relief of pain or fever, in doses appropriate for the child's age and weight. If the child is still suffering from symptoms more than forty-eight hours after antibiotic treatment has started, the child should be re-examined to determine if the antibiotic needs to be changed.

The use of antibiotics to treat ear infections has been questioned recently by those who argue that some ear infections, like colds, are caused by viruses rather than bacteria. Antibiotics are not effective in treating viruses. But in the case of otitis media, it's often impossible to determine whether the infection is caused by a virus or bacteria, or whether the infection will heal without the use of antibiotics. However, it is known that roughly one third of all ear infections do not heal on their own without the use of antibiotic treatment. Untreated otitis media has the potential to develop serious infectious complications if bacteria spread, including meningitis, infection to other bones in the ear, and, through the blood, to other areas of the body. It is because of these serious risks, antibiotic treatment is strongly recommended for most children less than three years of age with otitis media. For older children, the need for antibiotics depends on the individual situation.

## Consequences of Repeated Ear Infections

Recurrence of ear infections is not uncommon. In the vast majority of children, there will be some fluid present behind the eardrum following an ear infection, and it usually clears on its own. But in some cases, fluid in the middle ear persists for more than twelve weeks, even after the infection has cleared up. The presence of fluid behind the eardrum may interfere with transmission of sound; in other words, the fluid may cause a temporary reduction in hearing. If persistent fluid reduces a young child's hearing for an extended period of time, it may result in delayed language development and other problems. Also, if the fluid keeps getting infected, this results in recurrent or repeated ear infections.

## The Signs of Reduced Hearing in Children

With repeated infections, the child may show signs of reduced hearing. He may seem more inattentive, shout or speak loudly when talking, and sit closer to the television than he used to. Parents may find that they need to speak more loudly to the child in order to hold his attention. Another sign of reduced hearing in a very young child with recurring infections is that he or she is slower than other children in developing language skills.

## Detecting Fluid in the Middle Ear or a Hearing Problem

A physician can determine if there is persistent fluid by examining the eardrum with an otoscope; and/or by carrying out a special test called a tympanogram, which can identify the presence of fluid in the middle ear. Hearing can be assessed with a test called an audiogram. If these tests confirm that persistent middle ear fluid is causing reduced hearing, pressure equalization tubes (PE tubes) may be recommended for the child.

## About PE Tubes

PE tubes are inserted into the eardrum during a minor surgical procedure performed by an ENT specialist. This simple process is by far the most common type of surgery performed on children in North America. Before surgery, young children are usually given a mild general anesthetic, but older children may only need a local anesthetic. Most children are allowed to return home the same day as the surgery. Once the microscopic tube is inserted into the eardrum, fluid in the middle ear is able to drain through to the outside. As the fluid drains, the eardrum is once again able to vibrate normally, so hearing improves right away. The PE tube also helps prevent further infections. Since fluid drains to the outside, bacteria do not have a chance to multiply in fluid in the middle ear and cause infection.

# E. Coli Infections and Hamburger Disease

Also known as *Escherichia coli* , *E. coli* bacteria frequently cause diarrhea and other problems such as urinary tract infections. There are many types of *E. coli*. Some cause damage to the intestine, while others cause disease by a toxin they make. *E. coli* is found in the intestines of cows, contaminated soil, vegetation, water, and ground beef. People usually get infected by drinking contaminated water or eating uncooked contaminated meat or unwashed vegetables. The infection usually is limited to diarrhea with some blood in it and severe abdominal pain. However, certain strains are more dangerous and potentially deadly.

The *E. coli* O157 strain caused the outbreak in Walkerton, Ontario in May 2000 and is the germ behind Hamburger disease. *E. coli* O157 secretes a poisonous verotoxin. A serious complication in about 2 percent to 7 percent of infected people is Hemolytic Uremic Syndrome (HUS). HUS can occur within a week or two after the initial infection. In HUS, the *E. coli* toxins cause the red blood cells to break down, resulting in severe anemia. The toxins can also cause kidney failure, requiring dialysis. Unfortunately, HUS can cause death. Among the survivors, there can be a high rate of long-term complications. *E. coli* O157 strain complications typically occur in young children, the elderly, and persons with chronic medical conditions.

Although tests that identify these bacteria are available, there is no specific treatment. Prevention is our best defence. Here are some tips adapted from the Public Health Agency of Canada to prevent *E. coli* O157 infections:

- Thoroughly wash raw fruits and vegetables (including those with skins and rinds that aren't eaten) with clean, safe, running water before you prepare and eat them. Discard outer leaves of leafy vegetables before washing. Scrub fruits and vegetables that have firm surfaces such as oranges, melons, potatoes, and carrots, and cut away any damaged or bruised areas on produce.

- Do not store raw meats on a shelf above ready-to-eat foods in the refrigerator.
- Always cook meat to the proper temperature using a food thermometer and make sure that frozen hamburgers are well cooked, because they take longer to cook than room-temperature hamburgers.
- Be careful not to put cooked burgers on the same plate as raw burgers.
- Avoid unpasteurized juices and raw milk.
- Clean and disinfect all surfaces and utensils after use.
- Make sure that drinking water and the water you swim in is chlorinated and properly monitored.

# Eczema (Atopic Dermatitis)

Up to 20 percent of babies and young children have a skin condition called eczema, also known as atopic dermatitis. The eczema rash is scaly, red, itchy, and dry, and may appear during the first few weeks of age. In babies, the rash usually appears on the face, scalp, and on the outer areas of the arms and legs. In older children, it is in the creases of the elbows, knees, and wrists. Most children outgrow eczema, but in some cases, it may recur or persist into adulthood. When a child repeatedly scratches, this can lead to inflamed, rough, thickened skin. Babies and toddlers in particular are more susceptible to skin infection due to the constant scratching. The itchiness caused by eczema can be quite severe, and in some cases can lead to sleep disruption and family worry.

The exact cause of eczema is not known, but it often occurs with other allergic (atopic) conditions. Usually there is also a strong family history of atopic conditions, including respiratory and food allergies and /or asthma. Please note that **current evidence shows no link between a food allergy and eczema**. In other words, eating a certain food does not cause or worsen eczema.

## A Treatment Approach

The goals of treatment are to control inflammation and itching, and prevent infection. The most important part of the treatment is to keep the skin moist and well hydrated. This can be achieved by applying moisturizing creams regularly and by avoiding soaps that tend to dry the skin. In addition, after a bath, do not rub the skin dry with a towel, but rather gently pat it dry. It is also helpful to avoid woollen clothing, which can make eczema worse. Cotton clothing is better, preferably white, as the dye in coloured clothing may irritate the skin even more.

Depending on the situation, in addition to the above practical approaches, steroid creams or ointments or newer anti-inflammatory creams may be prescribed. Always use these preparations exactly as directed. In some situations to help alleviate the itchiness and allow baby to sleep, an antihistamine syrup may be prescribed as well.

# Failure to Thrive (Inadequate Weight Gain)

One of the most important parts of the routine pediatric checkup is to weigh and measure children in order to ensure that their growth is normal. Also, when evaluating children for any given problem, the pattern of weight gain is a key clue. When a parent is concerned that a child is not eating properly or is always sick, I first look at their weight gain. Regardless of the parental concern, it is reassuring if the weight gain is normal. Having said that, failure to thrive in children is something that we take very seriously.

## What Causes Failure to Thrive?

Although there are many possible causes, it really has to do with two basic elements: the amount of calories consumed and the amount of calories used or lost. Let me explain further. Depending on size and age, children need a certain daily amount of calories to grow normally. Obviously, if a child is not eating enough, the growth will be inadequate. On the other hand, a child may be ingesting enough for growth, but is losing the calories by not absorbing food well. This happens in children who have cystic fibrosis or other intestinal problems such as inflammatory bowel disease. Some children with inadequate weight gain have underlying conditions that cause them to burn more calories than normal. Such conditions include chronic lung problems, heart defects, and persistent urinary tract infections. Certain children with genetic abnormalities just seem to have a higher caloric need for their age.

When we evaluate a child with failure to thrive, we focus on the following:

- A calorie count, which is a detailed calculation of exactly how many calories per day a child is eating. Of course, in a young baby, this will also include an assessment of breastfeeding itself. For example, Is baby latching on properly? Is baby getting enough? or Is the mother producing enough milk?
- A complete physical assessment, which will include the necessary tests to diagnose any physical problem, anomaly, genetic abnormality, or infection.
- The family and social situation; children who are emotionally deprived can actually stop growing; this can be reversed by providing a loving family and social environment.

Most of the time, an underlying cause or problem is not found. However, for all children with failure to thrive, our goals are to achieve catch-up growth and to maintain normal weight gain subsequently.

The treatment team can consist of a variety of specialists including healthcare providers, dieticians, nurses, social workers, and psychologists. Which specialists get involved and whether the treatment and evaluation take place at home or in hospital depend on the individual situation and the severity of the growth delay.

The treatment for failure to thrive focuses on treating any associated conditions (if any) and ensuring adequate caloric intake, including supplementing with any necessary vitamins and minerals. Extra calories are provided by the addition of protein and carbohydrates to meals. Certain specially designed beverages or supplements can provide another important source of extra calories. These drinks contain all the necessary calories, as well as nutrients, vitamins, and supplements.

This can be a frustrating experience for all involved. However, with patience, proper caloric and nutritional supplementation, and the appropriate treatment and support from the various specialists, most children do begin to gain weight.

# Febrile Seizures

Febrile seizures are perhaps one of the scariest things that parents witness. Reassuringly, simple febrile seizures do not result in any brain damage or long-term intellectual consequences.

Febrile seizures occur in 3 percent of children, mostly between the ages of six months and five years. There may be a family tendency toward having febrile seizures. Experts suggest that, even though we do not know the exact cause of febrile seizures, they are due to immature brain wave activity in response to a sudden change of body temperature. So it is not the degree of the fever, but rather the rate at which it rises that may be a trigger.

Simple febrile seizures have the following characteristics:

- They are generalized; in other words, the whole body convulses or shakes.
- They last less than fifteen minutes.
- They occur only once within a twenty-four-hour period.
- The child has a normal development.
- There is no history of seizures in the absence of a fever in the child and in the family.
- There is no infection of the nervous system (such as meningitis).

The key in evaluating a child who has had a febrile seizure is making sure that it is a typical or simple febrile seizure, and that the convulsions were not due to any other factors. Accordingly, blood tests or even a lumbar puncture may be performed to make sure that there is nothing else going on. Once we are certain that it is a typical febrile seizure, we want to find the cause of the fever, and if it's bacterial, treat it with the appropriate antibiotics. In most cases, it is usually of viral origin. An

EEG (an electroencephalogram) may be performed six weeks later to make sure there is no brain wave seizure or epileptic abnormality.

Once a child has had a confirmed febrile seizure, parents want to know if it will recur. The chance of a child having another febrile seizure in the future is age-dependent. Children less than twelve months have a 50 percent chance of recurrent febrile seizures. In children older than one year, the recurrence rate is 30 percent.

## Will A Child With Febrile Seizures Develop Epilepsy?

Epilepsy is a seizure disorder in which a person convulses for no apparent reason. The risk for developing epilepsy in children who have had a simple febrile seizure is just a bit higher than 1 percent (the risk is 1 percent in the general population). In children who have their first seizure before twelve months of age and have had multiple simple febrile seizures, the risk for developing epilepsy by adulthood is 2.4 percent. The good news is that almost 98 percent of these children will not develop epilepsy.

## Preventing Febrile Seizures

There is no specific treatment for preventing febrile seizures. Anticonvulsive (anti-seizure) medications do not prevent febrile seizures. In certain cases where the seizures are prolonged or very recurrent, sedative-type medications may be helpful. Although anti-fever medications can help lower a fever, they do not prevent febrile seizures. If your child has had a febrile seizure, your healthcare provider will give you specific directions on what to do during future episodes of illness with fever.

# Fever

Normal body temperature is usually 37° Celsius (98.6° Fahrenheit). Whether a child is said to have a fever depends on how the temperature is taken. The child is considered to have a fever if the temperature is over the following readings:

- 38° C (100.4° F) rectally;
- 37.8° C (100° F) orally; or
- 37.2° C (99° F) in the axilla (armpit).

Fever is a symptom and not a diagnosis or a medical condition. The most common cause of a fever in children is an infection, mostly viral, but in some cases bacterial. One of the challenges in evaluating children with fever is trying to determine the cause, or at least to make sure it is not due a bacterial infection. This distinction is important, as viral infections do not need antibiotic treatment, but bacterial infections usually do. More rarely, there are other so called noninfectious causes of fever, but in these circumstances, fever persists for prolonged periods of time (weeks or even months), rather than just for a short period like with a current infection.

In general, the younger the child, the sicker-looking the child, and/or the longer the fever has persisted, the higher the chance of a bacterial infection. Also, as important as the degree of fever, is how a febrile child generally looks. A sick-looking child with a low fever may be more ill than a very well looking, active child with a higher fever.

## Taking a Child's Temperature

There are three ways to take a child's temperature:

- Rectally: this is the most exact reading and is recommended for children less than five years of age.
- Orally (by mouth): this is recommended for children older than five years of age
- Via the axilla (armpit): this is the least precise way to measure body temperature.

## Normal Body Temperature

The average (normal) body temperature is usually 37° C (98.6° F) rectally. However, there are ranges of normal temperature depending on how it is measured:

- When measured rectally it is between 36.6° C and 38° C (or 97.9° F and 100.4° F);
- When taken by mouth it is between 35.5° C and 37.5° C (or 95.9° F and 99.5° F);
- When taken at the armpit it is between 34.7° C and 37.3° C (or 94.5° F and 99.1° F).

## What Is Considered To Be Fever?

A child is considered to have a fever if:

- The rectal temperature is greater than 38° C (or 100.4° F);
- The oral temperature is greater than 37.8° C (or 100° F);
- The armpit temperature is greater than 37.2° C (or 99° F).

## Fever Medications

Today, there are two commonly used anti-fever (antipyretic) medications:

- Acetaminophen (sold under the labels Tylenol®, Tempra®, and Panadol®) is a medication that has a long and favourable track record and is considered to be appropriate for use in children for fever and/or pain control. Available in liquid, drop, or pill form, acetaminophen is given every four to six hours as needed. Acetaminophen is also available in suppository form, which can be helpful when a child needs to take fever medication but is throwing up, with a gastrointestinal infection. Although acetaminophen is considered safe when used as recommended, taking it regularly for more than a week at a time can be dangerous. Overdosing with acetaminophen can result in liver damage. So it is important to follow the dosage based on a child's age or weight and not to give it regularly for more than four or five days.
- Ibuprofen (sold under the labels Advil® and Motrin®) is a fever medication that is newer than acetaminophen. Most experts agree that ibuprofen is a relatively safe and very effective medication, but I still usually recommend acetaminophen as a first line fever medication, given its longer track record.

## Using Fever Medications in Children

- Aspirin (acetylsalicylic acid—ASA) should never be used in children. When given with certain viral infections including chickenpox and influenza, ASA has been associated with a sometimes fatal condition called Reye's syndrome that can result in liver and brain damage.
- Overdosing by accidental ingestion of these fever medications can be very serious. These medications, as with all others, should be stored well out of the reach of children.
- Acetaminophen and ibuprofen are available in combined preparations with decongestants and/or cough medicines. These combination forms should be avoided.

- If a child is on antibiotics for a bacterial infection (for example, an ear infection) and has fever, then fever medication can be given as well for temperature control during the first forty-eight hours. This is the time usually needed for antibiotics to start working.

## Other Measures to Help Lower the Fever

Lowering the temperature with acetaminophen or ibuprofen can help your child feel better and be less irritable. It usually takes between sixty and ninety minutes for the fever to go down. If fever medication does not bring the temperature down, the child could be given a lukewarm sponge bath. Do not use cool or cold compresses or baths and never use alcohol sponging. Also, children with fever should not be overdressed.

## When to Call Your Healthcare Provider

Worrisome or alarm signs needing immediate medical attention include:

- The child with the fever is less than three months of age.
- The fever is higher than 39.5° C (103° F) rectally;
- The child appears unwell or unusually ill (this applies even when there is no fever);
- Persistent fever (more than three to four days).

## Fifth Disease

Fifth disease (or *erythema infectiosum*) is caused by a virus called parvovirus B19. The name "fifth disease" is derived from the fact that was the fifth childhood infection with rash that was discovered. Fifth disease is most common in children aged between five and fifteen years old and begins with a low-grade fever, headache, and mild cold-like symptoms. A few days later, a bright red rash develops on the face, giving a slapped-cheek appearance. The net-like or lacy rash then spreads to the trunk, arms, and legs. It may take up to three weeks for the rash to completely clear. In the meantime, exposure to sunlight, heat, exercise, and stress may worsen the rash. Rarely, mostly in older kids and adults, the parvovirus infection may cause hand, wrist, knee, and ankle joint swelling or pain.

The vast majority of people who develop fifth disease get over the infection without any consequences or complications. However, children with weakened immune systems (e.g. AIDS) or certain blood disorders (e.g. sickle-cell anemia) may become quite ill. Also, parvovirus B19 infection during pregnancy may cause problems for the unborn child, especially if the infection occurs during the first half of the pregnancy. Fortunately, about 50 percent of all pregnant women are immune or protected, having had a previous infection with parvovirus. Serious problems occur in less than 5 percent of women who become infected during pregnancy. Female teachers and child caregivers of child-bearing age should be aware of this potential complication. Pregnant women who develop a rash or have been exposed to someone with fifth disease should call their obstetrician.

Making the diagnosis of fifth disease usually rests upon recognizing the characteristic rash a child develops. Specific blood tests are also available to determine if a child is infected by the parvovirus. These same tests are used to determine if someone has had a parvovirus infection in the past. This would be important if we wanted to determine whether, for example, a pregnant woman in contact with fifth disease is immune or not. If the blood test shows that she has had parvovirus infection in the past, then she is protected.

## Fifth Disease Treatment

There are no available antiviral medications that will treat fifth disease; nor can it be treated with antibiotics. Usually, children with fifth disease feel fairly well and need little treatment other than rest. Acetaminophen (Tylenol®, Tempra®, and Panadol®) may be recommended for fever or joint pain. At this time, there is no vaccine for fifth disease.

## When Is a Parvovirus Infection Contagious?

A child with fifth disease is most contagious a few days before the rash appears. Note that a child is usually not contagious once the rash appears . Isolating a child with a fifth disease rash will not prevent spread of the infection because the child usually is not contagious by that time.

# Food Allergies

Whether or not food allergies are on the rise is uncertain, but our awareness of their existence and potential danger has increased over the last decade.

## What Is an Allergy?

An allergy is the body's reaction to a certain substance, which is then known as an allergen. This substance can enter the body through ingestion, inhalation, or contact with the skin. An allergic reaction is caused by the body's immune system. While there are different types of allergic reactions, as far as food is concerned, the ones that we are most concerned about are the immediate, generalized reactions. Symptoms of such an allergic reaction include:

- Difficulty breathing with or without wheezing;
- Swollen throat or tongue;
- Swelling, especially around the face and mouth;
- A rash or hives, also known as urticaria;
- Low blood pressure;
- Heart failure;
- Nausea and vomiting;
- Cramps and diarrhea;
- Loss of consciousness.

These generalized reactions are referred to as anaphylaxis, which unfortunately can be deadly. However, these symptoms can be due to other problems. For example, cramps, diarrhea, and vomiting can occur as a result of food poisoning, rather than a food allergy. An asthma attack (wheezing and difficulty breathing) on its own is not usually due to an immediate food allergy. Note that an anaphylactic (general) reaction usually occurs within ninety minutes of ingesting the food to which a child is allergic.

If your child has ever had any one of these symptoms within a short time of eating a particular food, you should discuss this with a healthcare provider. Of course, in an emergency, seek immediate, urgent medical aid.

## Common Causes of Food Allergy

While theoretically any food can cause an allergy, the following are the most common allergens for children:

- Cow's milk is the most common food allergy in young children. Please read the chapter on Cow's Milk Protein Allergy;
- Soya;
- Eggs;
- Peanuts;
- Nuts;
- Wheat;
- Seafood.

Importantly, sulfites, other preservatives, and artificial food colorants (food dyes) can also cause allergic reactions.

## How Is a Food Allergy Confirmed?

A simple skin test (see the information on allergy tests in the chapter entitled, Allergies and Testing) or blood test can confirm the presence of an allergy. Once an allergy has been confirmed and the physician feels that there is a potential for future anaphylactic reactions, the parents are told to strictly avoid that food.

In such cases, the doctor will prescribe medications to keep on hand in case of an accidental ingestion of the food the child is allergic to. This may be an antihistamine syrup and in many situations, an auto injector, which looks like a pen but contains a pre-measured amount of adrenaline (also known as epinephrine). Adrenaline is the only medication that can reverse or stop an anaphylactic reaction and administering it immediately can save lives.

One such injector is called EpiPen® and is to be with the child wherever she goes. Today, most schools have an EpiPen® (or similar injector) on hand and are quite familiar with how to use one. If a child ever requires her EpiPen®, emergency transportation to the nearest hospital should immediately follow at all times. Note that once the EpiPen® or similar auto injector is used, its effect will only last about thirty minutes. So if you live farther than thirty minutes away from your nearest hospital, you will need more than one EpiPen® on hand. Your allergist will provide you with specific details relevant to your situation.

Other types of reactions may occur as a result of eating foods, including intolerances and other symptoms that are neither allergy-based, nor life-threatening. This is why it is important to evaluate a child with a suspected food allergy to identify and confirm an allergy so the necessary avoidance precautions are taken. On the other hand, in the case of an allergy not being found, restricting the child's diet is not necessary.

Some food allergies are outgrown, for example, milk and egg allergies and even peanut allergies (in a small percentage of children). The age at which a child can outgrow an allergy depends on the type of food and individual circumstances. If your child has a proven or known food allergy, never try to give the child that food to see whether he still has the allergy or whether he has outgrown it. Before attempting to introduce that particular food, it is absolutely necessary to have a medical re-evaluation of your child, which includes another skin test and possibly a blood test. Only after retesting can your allergist be in a position to advise you whether or not to retry that particular food. In some cases, a food challenge may be needed. This is where the child will be given the food to eat as a test, but in a hospital or clinic setting that is equipped and ready to treat any allergic reactions should they occur.

# Gastroenteritis: Diarrhea and Vomiting

Gastroenteritis is an infection of the gastrointestinal system; in other words, an infection of the stomach and/or the intestines. Sometimes it is referred to as the stomach flu or as gastro. Note that stomach flu is unrelated to the flu caused by the influenza virus. The symptoms usually include diarrhea and/or vomiting, one or the other, or both at the same time. There may also be associated low-grade fever, abdominal pain, or cramps. In most cases, the illness lasts for three to six days. Often, there is a history of contact with a person who has had similar symptoms.

## What Causes Gastroenteritis?

There are many possible causes of gastroenteritis in children, but the most common are viruses such as the rotavirus, which tends to infect younger children. This is why most children with diarrhea get better on their own, without any specific medications or antibiotics. Some viruses cause symptoms of gastroenteritis only, while others can also cause cold symptoms. Other causes include bacterial infections as well as certain parasites like giardia or amoebas.

### Norwalk Virus

Another virus commonly associated with outbreaks of gastroenteritis is the Norwalk virus. First discovered in Norwalk, Ohio, this virus has been at the root of several epidemics or outbreaks of gastroenteritis across North America in hospital emergency rooms, schools, and even on cruise ships. There is a group of similar or related viruses that are referred to as Norwalk-like viruses or agents. These viruses can infect people of any age and usually cause profuse watery diarrhea, vomiting, and fatigue. The infection lasts a few days and there is no specific treatment. Most of the time, it spreads from one person to another through direct or indirect contact with infected feces or vomit. The virus is highly infectious and tends to occur in clusters, like in a school and in hospital wards. More rarely, it can also be transmitted by drinking water that contains the virus, or by eating food contaminated by this virus. The infection develops within one to two days after contact with an infected person or substance.

### Rotavirus

The rotavirus is the most common cause of serious gastroenteritis in babies and children less than two years of age. The symptoms and complications are the same as described above. The reason I mention this virus is that there is now a vaccine for Rotavirus, given by mouth to infants less than six months of age. This vaccine has been shown to be effective in preventing this infection in young babies who are at high risk for dehydration and the need for hospitalization from gastroenteritis.

### Bacterial Causes of Gastroenteritis

Less commonly, several different types of bacteria can also cause gastroenteritis. Importantly, food poisoning is a form of gastroenteritis that can occur if a person eats or drinks contaminated (spoiled) food or water. This is why—in order to prevent food poisoning—it is necessary to cook foods well and to make sure that they are properly refrigerated.

## Treating Gastroenteritis

The main concern when dealing with diarrhea (and/or vomiting) is dehydration and trying to prevent it as much as best as possible. Children, especially young babies and infants can easily become dehydrated if they lose more fluid than they take in, which can be quite dangerous. So taking care of them is like playing catch-up, with the goal being for them to drink enough fluids to make up for the fluid lost in the diarrhea and/or vomiting.

Fortunately, in most cases, the treatment is simply to give the child adequate amounts of fluid, depending on the severity of the symptoms. Recently, healthcare providers have modified their approach to treating mild cases of diarrhea and usually do not change the child's diet at all. In moderate illness, specific liquids are used, called oral rehydration solutions. Never give only water to a child who is vomiting or has diarrhea. This can be dangerous. The body needs specific amounts of salt and sugar, which are not in adequate amounts in water nor in watered-down juices and soft drinks. Only oral rehydration solutions such as Pedialyte® and Infalyte® contain the right amounts of sugar and salt. Generally, milk can be continued as long as it does not make the diarrhea worse. Breastfeeding can usually continue as well. Also, if a child is hungry, let him eat.

If a child has just vomited, parents should wait for half an hour and then begin giving fluids starting with one tablespoon. If the child keeps that down, five minutes later, one and a half tablespoons can be given, and so on, progressively increasing the amount each time by adding another half a tablespoon every five to ten minutes. Should the child vomit again, take a break for about thirty minutes and start the cycle over again. If the child cannot keep any fluids down, medical attention should be sought. Happily, most children will be able to keep down enough fluid, and the vomiting—as well as any other associated gastroenteritis symptoms—will go away on its own. If a vomiting child also has a fever and cannot keep the fever medication down, suppository acetaminophen is a very practical solution.

Most cases of diarrhea are caused by viruses, which are not treated by antibiotics. In certain cases of bacterial infection, antibiotics may be prescribed, depending on the individual situation, the age of the child, and the specific type of bacteria causing the infection. In addition, if the cause is a parasite (very rare in North America), anti-parasitic medications are prescribed.

Note that anti-diarrheal medicines should not be used in children. They are not helpful and indeed may be harmful.

## Protracted Diarrhea Of Childhood

In the past, most children with diarrhea would be fed a very bland diet for prolonged periods. This approach actually made matters worse. Modern medicine has now come to recognize a condition called Protracted Diarrhea of Childhood. Children suffering from this condition have diarrhea that simply will not go away and they needed to be admitted to hospital for weeks or even months of intravenous therapy. They might have started off with a simple or typical viral-induced diarrhea, which just seemed to get worse. It is now understood that this protracted diarrhea is due to the fact that these children were being given low-calorie diets. Because the intestinal lining did not get enough nutrition, it became damaged and started to leak, allowing liquids into the intestine, causing large amounts of diarrhea. This is why current recommendations stipulate that, aside from the use of appropriate oral rehydration solutions, a normal diet should resume as soon as possible. Consequently, the so-called BRAT diet of banana, rice, apple sauce, and toast, which are low in both calories and fats, should not be used for prolonged periods of time (no more than a day or two) if at all.

## Signs of Dehydration

In babies and young children, the signs of dehydration include:

- Less frequent urination (less than six wet diapers per day, in babies);
- No tears when crying;
- Dry or sticky mouth;

- Weight loss;
- Extreme thirst.

## When Should a Healthcare Provider Be Consulted?

Take your child to a healthcare provider immediately if any of the following symptoms are present:

- There are signs of dehydration;
- Your baby is younger than three months;
- There is blood in the stool;
- There is frequent vomiting preventing her from drinking;
- The diarrhea lasts for more than one week;
- Your child complains of abdominal pain, looks or behaves unwell and/or has high fever.

Severe cases of diarrhea and/or vomiting and dehydration are relatively rare. The only treatment is the administration of intravenous fluids in a hospital setting. Because each child is different, treatment is based on the individual situation.

## Are Special Tests Needed?

In most children with diarrhea, stool tests or other tests are not necessary. However, if a physician suspects bacteria as the cause, then a stool culture (a test for bacteria or parasites) will be collected and sent for laboratory testing.

## Prevention

The prevention approach for gastroenteritis is hand washing before and after contact with any infected individual, and decontamination of areas such as toilets, sinks, and other objects that might have come in contact with infected stool or vomit.

# Gastroesophageal Reflux Disease (GERD)

As described in a previous section of this book, more than 40 percent of normal babies spit-up (also known as regurgitating). This is due to an immature sphincter (a muscle like an elastic band) that is too weak to control exit from a baby's stomach. Because the sphincter is not mature and not working well, contents of the stomach are pushed back up into the esophagus or all the way up to the mouth as the stomach contracts to digest the food. When there are no health consequences, this is known as simple spitting- up or Gastroesophageal Reflux (GER). However, when there are associated health consequences, it is referred to as Gastroesophageal Reflux Disease (GERD).

## The Two General Categories of GERD

### Visible GERD

A baby spits up so much that not only is it visible, but, unlike simple GER, it prevents normal weight gain and growth.

### Invisible or Not-So-Obvious GERD

The reflux of the stomach contents do not travel all the way up to the mouth. They go up only into the esophagus or to the back of the throat (larynx). This non-regurgitant form of reflux can certainly cause health problems. Esophagitis is an irritation of the esophagus caused by the acid that refluxes back up. The symptoms are like heartburn, and in babies it usually is pain and crying while feeding. Reflux contents in the esophagus and throat area can also cause apnea, cough, and worsen asthma symptoms (even without obvious GERD signs).

## Tests for GERD

When we suspect that a baby's regurgitation prevents weight gain, special X-rays can confirm the reflux and its extent. In other situations where there is no obvious vomiting or spitting up, and GERD is suspected, a specific test called a pH Probe can measure the acidity level in the esophagus. Normally, there should be no acid in the esophagus and if there is, it confirms reflux. In some situations, as part of evaluating babies with apnea, asthma, or cough, testing for GERD may be done.

## Treating GERD

There are several treatment approaches for GERD, including the use of prescribed medications that reduce the stomach acid level or help with stomach movement (motility). Very rarely, in severe cases of visible regurgitation causing significant growth delay or failure to gain weight, surgical repair may be required. The specific type of treatment approach depends on the individual situation.

# Hand, Foot, and Mouth Disease

Hand, foot, and mouth disease occurs primarily during the summer and fall months and is caused by a type of enterovirus. Enteroviruses are a group of viruses that cause a large variety of rashes and infections. As a matter of fact, during the summer and fall months, these viruses are the most common causes of viral rashes in children. It is also interesting that the younger a child, the more likely she will develop a rash as a result of infection from these viruses. Older individuals may get the infection, but their symptoms are less severe and nonspecific—just a bit of fever or a bit of diarrhea.

Among the group of enteroviruses are various specific viruses including the coxsackievirus and echovirus. Each group has different subtypes, which are classified based on a number. For example, the coxsackievirus A16 strain is the major cause of hand, foot, and mouth disease.

## Symptoms of Hand, Foot, and Mouth Disease

Typically, there are small lesions or spots inside the mouth, mostly on the tongue, and inside the inner front part of the mouth, known as the buccal mucosa. Additionally, a rash develops on the hands and the feet. It is described as being vesicular, looking as though it has a bit of fluid in its centre.

There can be fever and other symptoms too, including abdominal pain, vomiting, and diarrhea. The diagnosis is usually easy to make, due to the very characteristic location of the rash and the summer or fall seasonal occurrence of the infection. The infection can last for up to one week and usually goes away on its own without any specific treatment. The virus spreads from one person to another by contact, for example from the hands of an infected person. So prevention is best practised by washing hands thoroughly when in contact with a person infected with this or any other enteroviral infection. Once a person has come into contact with the virus, it takes about four to six days for the infection to show itself; this is called the incubation period.

## Other Summertime Infections

Some enteroviruses can cause an infection with or without a rash. For example, echovirus 9 causes a total body rash and fever. Other enteroviruses can cause a variety of symptoms including isolated fever, abdominal pain, vomiting, and diarrhea. Often, there are outbreaks of these types of infections in daycare centres, summer sleep-away camps, and day camps. Again, these infections go away on their own without any specific treatment. It is important to make sure that a child who is vomiting and/or has diarrhea does not become dehydrated by ensuring that he keeps drinking the appropriate fluids.

Aseptic or viral meningitis can also be caused by certain enteroviruses. This type of meningitis again occurs mostly during the summer and resolves on its own. Fortunately, contrary to bacterial meningitis, viral meningitis usually has no complications or consequences.

# Head Lice

Head lice infestation (also known as pediculosis), one of the most common contagious childhood diseases, is caused by barely visible insects found almost exclusively on the human scalp. Contrary to popular belief, head lice infestation has little to do with personal hygiene. In fact, head lice are totally non-discriminating, and can infest people of any lifestyle, age, race, or socioeconomic status, since lice multiply and spread quickly from person to person.

## Head Lice Appearance and Growth

Head lice are greyish in colour and barely visible to the naked eye. Identifying lice can be difficult as they move very rapidly upon six legs. Lice require warmth and humidity to survive, and so they tend to be most concentrated around the back of the host's head and behind the ears. A single female may lay up to 150 eggs (also known as nits), during her lifetime. Nits are silvery-white in colour, oval in shape, and may look to the naked eye like tiny grains of sand cemented to the hair shaft. Nits are smaller than adult lice, but are generally easier to identify, because they're more numerous and don't move. Seven to nine days after being laid, the nits hatch and give birth to young lice who then start their own life cycles.

## Common Questions About Lice Transmission

**Question:** Is the presence of lice a sign of poor personal hygiene?
**Answer:** No. Head lice seem to prefer a clean scalp and, otherwise, show no particular preference for a human host's sex, race, age, cleanliness, or socioeconomic status.
**Question:** Are only children susceptible?

**Answer:** No. Lice show no preference for children over adults. However, infestation is more common among children between the age of three and ten years, because of their tendency to be in close contact with others—especially at school and daycares, on buses, in camps and playgrounds.

**Question:** Does long hair encourage infestation?

**Answer:** No. Since head lice are only interested in the immediate area of the scalp, cutting the hair will neither prevent nor alleviate infestation.

**Question:** Can lice be contracted from plants, animals, and pets?

**Answer:** No. Humans are the only hosts on which head lice survive. Head lice cannot live on animals, pets, or plants.

**Question:** Can lice jump or fly from one person to another?

**Answer:** Head lice have no wings; they can only crawl—so transmission comes only from direct contact with other infested people or their belongings. Indirect transmission can occur through sharing personal articles that come in contact with the scalp, such as hats, scarves, hair accessories, headgear, headphones, brushes, and combs.

## How Is Head Lice Infestation Detected?

The main symptoms of a head lice infestation are itching and irritation of the scalp. Itching is usually persistent and more intense during the night. Head lice infestation can be diagnosed by confirming the presence of living lice or viable nits on the head. They are visible to the naked eye, or with the use of a magnifying glass. Although nits are generally easier to detect than lice, they can be confused with specks of dandruff, skin debris, or hair product residue. This mistake can be avoided by testing the adhesiveness of the specks to the hair shaft. Unlike other substances, nits cannot be removed easily with fingernails or by washing the hair.

It's important to be aware that the mere presence of nits in the hair does not necessarily indicate a current head lice infestation.

## What Happens if Lice Are Found on a Child?

If living head lice or viable nits are found on a student, the school authorities usually send the infested child home with a letter to the child's parents, explaining what the problem is and suggesting that the child see a pharmacist or physician for treatment. Parents and children are usually assured that they are not to blame for head lice infestation, that there's no need for panic, anxiety, or embarrassment, and that the problem can be resolved quickly and effectively with the proper treatment and precautionary measures.

If more than one student is found to have head pediculosis, a sample of children from each grade should be examined by the nurse in order to estimate the degree of the outbreak. If the infestation becomes difficult to control, the nurse may need assistance from the local public health department to fully evaluate and control the problem.

## How Are Head Lice Infestations Treated?

There are three important treatment components:

### Pediculicidal Treatment

A variety of pediculicidal treatments is available in the form of shampoos, cream rinses, and aerosols. Properly administered, the application usually kills all lice, though some nits may survive. Most pediculicidal treatments require a second application after a given period of time, in order to wipe out any lice that may have hatched from surviving nits. The specific treatment should be discussed with the child's healthcare provider, nurse, or pharmacist. For successful treatment, instructions for how to use the product must be strictly adhered to. Misuse or repeated dosages of pediculicides can render treatment ineffective, make the problem worse, or even cause harm.

### Use of a Fine-Toothed Comb

The use of a special comb to remove nits and head lice after application of a pediculicide is essential to successfully completing treatment. Immediately after rinsing the pediculicide from the hair, the fine-toothed comb should be used on one small lock of hair at a time, combing toward the scalp and then back, to remove all nits and lice. This operation should take about two hours and requires a great deal of patience, but must be done in order to avoid reinfestation.

### Disinfection of Exposed Items

Head lice can live for about forty-eight hours away from the host, while nits can survive for up to two weeks. So another important precaution for preventing reinfestation (or infestation of other family members) involves the disinfection of personal articles and other items that are likely to have come into contact with the scalp. These may include hats, scarves, hair accessories, towels, and bedding items. Clothing that may have come in contact with the patient's hair should be washed in very hot water and dried in the hottest cycle of the dryer for at least twenty minutes. The same should be done for towels and bedding items. Brushes and combs can be disinfected by soaking in hot water for ten minutes. Items that cannot be washed should be either dry-cleaned, ironed with a hot iron, or sealed in a plastic bag for two weeks.

## What About Family and Other Close Contacts?

In order to reduce chances of reinfestation and to control the outbreak of head lice, it's important that anyone who's been in close contact with the infested person—whether family members, schoolmates, or friends—be informed, examined, and if necessary, treated. Any other infested individuals should be treated at the same time.

# Hepatitis A and B

## Hepatitis A

The hepatitis A virus (HAV) is one that infects the liver and is spread through water and food. It is usually present under conditions of a poor water supply, poor hygiene, and poor sanitation. The word "hepatitis" means inflammation of the liver. The virus is spread from person to person by the fecal-oral route, in other words, through contact with infected people, either directly or indirectly, by eating contaminated food or water. Young children are able to infect other children or family members.

## Symptoms of Hepatitis A

Usually, it takes between fifteen and fifty days for the infection to develop after initial contact (the incubation period); symptoms can last about four to six weeks. The symptoms of HAV infection include:

- Fever;
- Weakness;
- Fatigue;
- Loss of appetite;
- Nausea;
- Abdominal pain;
- Jaundice (yellow skin and eyes).

The symptoms can range from mild (lasting up to two weeks) to severe (lasting several months). In areas where HAV is very common (endemic), most HAV infections occur in young children. Specific blood tests can confirm the diagnosis of HAV. There is no specific treatment or medication. However, some people may require hospitalization for dehydration and other supportive treatments such as intravenous (IV) fluids.

## Preventing Hepatitis A

From the community point of view, good sanitation and a clean water supply prevents the spread of HAV. Personal hygiene, including hand washing especially before and after all meals, is a very important measure. Fortunately, there is also a vaccine available for HAV. This vaccine requires an initial dose and then a booster (a second shot) between six to twelve months later. The booster dose ensures protection for up to twenty years. This is recommended for travellers planning to visit countries where there is poor sanitation and HAV infections are frequent. There is a hepatitis vaccine that protects against both HAV and hepatitis B. Your healthcare provider can give you more details.

## Hepatitis B

A hepatitis B infection, also known as serum hepatitis, is an infection of the liver caused by the hepatitis B virus, a **dangerous, but preventable infection**. In North America, hepatitis B occurs mostly in adolescents and young adults, although anyone can become infected.

The infection is usually silent, without any apparent symptoms for many years. One of the most serious complications of hepatitis B is liver cancer or irreparable liver damage or failure. In general, the earlier in life one is infected, the higher the chances that these complications develop. Not all people with the infection will be sick or have any symptoms; they are referred to as hepatitis B carriers. Although not apparently ill, carriers may unknowingly transmit the virus to other people. The only way to know if you are a carrier is by a blood test.

## How is Hepatitis B Spread?

Hepatitis B can be transmitted from coming into contact with an infected person's blood or body fluids. Modes of transmission of hepatitis B include being passed from the mother to her baby at birth and living in the same household with someone who is infected, including a carrier. The virus can also be transmitted through unprotected sexual contact, or through contact with infected blood such as blood from drug users or others who share dirty tattoo needles or ear/body-piercing needles, and by sharing toothbrushes or razors.

There is no cure for hepatitis B infection, so prevention is extremely important. Thanks to the hepatitis B vaccine, over 95 percent of vaccinated children are protected from the infection. The hepatitis B vaccination is currently part of the regular immunization schedule in North America. The vaccination consists of two or three doses. All doses should be given for maximal protection. In order to protect children and adolescents who have not previously received the vaccination, hepatitis B vaccine is recommended at age ten to twelve. Older adolescents or others living with an infected household member should also receive the vaccination series. In high-risk areas or situations, the vaccination is given during the newborn period. Your healthcare provider or local public health agency will give you the specific details and counsel you on what is best for your baby in your region.

Aside from hepatitis B vaccination, another important aspect of prevention focuses on avoiding contact with infected blood. By knowing and avoiding potentially high-risk behaviours. Using condoms during sexual intercourse, and not sharing needles, razors, and toothbrushes can all help prevent the spread of the virus. Pregnant women should be tested for hepatitis B because, if they are infected, immediate action can be taken at birth to protect their newborn baby.

Finally, be aware that you are at a higher risk when travelling to China and some parts of Asia and Africa where the incidence of hepatitis B is higher than in North America.

## Hepatitis A and Hepatitis B Features

There are some common features shared by both these infections:

- Both are viruses.
- Both hepatitis A and B infect the liver.
- There is no treatment for either.
- Vaccines are available against both of these viruses.

However, there are some very important differences:

- HAV is spread by ingesting contaminated food or water. The hepatitis B virus is spread through blood-to-blood contact, such as through unprotected sex, blood transfusions, being passed from mother to baby at birth, and by sharing needles, razors, and toothbrushes.
- The HAV infection usually resolves its own, with no long-term consequences.
- Hepatitis B infection, on the other hand, is much more severe, as it can last permanently in various forms. Unfortunately, this can lead to liver failure and even liver cancer.

## Hernias

A hernia is a condition that some children are born with that literally is a piece of intestine that sticks out through a small hole in the abdominal muscle wall. A hernia can develop in the first few months after the baby is born because of a weakness in the muscles of the abdomen. Note that straining during a bowel movement and crying do not cause hernias. However, the increased pressure these actions produce on the abdomen can make a hernia more noticeable; it can be seen visibly bulging. The reason we worry about some types of hernias is that there is a risk that the intestine could twist on itself and cause problems that can lead to damaged intestines.

### Types of Hernias Seen In Babies and Infants

#### Inguinal Hernias

Inguinal hernias are found in the groin—the inguinal area. They tend to be more common in premature babies. Although these hernias occur mostly in boys, they can occur in girls as well, but much less frequently. Because of the risk of twisting and damaging the intestines, inguinal hernias require surgery to repair them. Each situation is different, but in general, it is recommended that they be repaired as soon possible after they are discovered. Hernia repair operations are performed under general anesthesia and usually in day surgery.

#### Umbilical Hernias

Umbilical hernias are sometimes referred as outies—the belly button pops outwards. They range in size from very small to very large, in fact, scaring many parents. Reassuringly, even the very big ones go away on their own with time.

The questions of how and when to treat umbilical hernias have been the source of debate for years. As a matter of fact, the so-called outie belly button is actually a small umbilical hernia that causes no problems even in adulthood. It is also interesting to know that Afro-American children are more prone to umbilical hernias, as are babies born prematurely or with a low birth-weight. In all these cases, as long as the hernia is shrinking and not giving the baby any discomfort, no treatment is necessary.

In the past, some umbilical hernias were treated by strapping. Strapping consists of wrapping a belt-like cloth around the waist at the level of the belly button to push the hernia back in. Sometimes, a coin is used as well. Today, strapping (with or without a coin) is considered ineffective and is not recommended.

Most (even very large) umbilical hernias will go away on their own by the age of five or six. Unlike the case of inguinal hernias, surgical repair of umbilical hernias is not routinely needed unless the intestines twist (this happens very rarely), the hernia persists beyond four or five years of age, or it starts to grow after the first or second year of life. This of course depends on the individual situation.

# Influenza Infection ... The Flu

## Is the Flu the Same as a Cold?

The answer to this question is no. The terms "a cold" and "the flu" refer to different things. The common cold, caused by any one of 250 viruses, lasts for a few days and causes a cough and a stuffy or runny nose, maybe accompanied by a fever. The flu, which is caused by the influenza virus, is potentially a more serious infection. The flu often begins like a cold, but is usually associated with the following:

- High fever;
- Severe muscle and body aches;
- Chills;
- A headache;
- Loss of appetite;
- Extreme fatigue; and
- Weakness.

While a cold usually lasts for a few days and goes away on its own without any complication or problem, the flu can last between seven and ten days or even longer. Also, the cough and fatigue from an influenza infection can persist for weeks.

**The bottom line is that the flu is not the same as a cold; it is potentially a much more dangerous infection than the common cold.**

## How Is the Flu Spread?

The influenza virus is spread from one person to another by airborne droplets in a cough or a sneeze. It is important to realize that the influenza virus can also be spread indirectly, because it can live for up forty-eight hours outside the body. Thus, this virus can be contracted from surfaces such as telephones, computer keyboards, doorknobs, and toys. Don't forget that unwashed hands and unwashed kitchen utensils can also transmit the virus.

## Who Is at Risk?

In children less than twenty-four months of age or children of any age with chronic medical conditions such as asthma, heart problems, or cystic fibrosis, an influenza infection can be complicated by serious and potentially deadly complications such as pneumonia. The influenza virus weakens the body's defence system and makes it easier for other infections to occur.

## Children and the Flu

Influenza infection rates are higher in younger children, and even healthy kids can end up quite sick as a result of the flu. Studies have shown that up to 42 percent of pre-school-age children develop the flu. In addition, during the influenza season, there are higher rates of ear infections, as well as severe bacterial lung infections among children.

## Treating the Flu

Unfortunately, there is no specific cure or medicine for the flu. There are some newer anti-influenza virus medications on the market, but they are not indicated for children. The best approach is prevention, which can be achieved by getting a flu vaccine. If a child develops the flu, the treatment includes the following:

- Rest;
- Drinking plenty of fluids;
- Acetaminophen (Tempra®, Children's Tylenol®, or Panadol®) for fever and pain.

## Some Important Points

Antibiotics are not effective against the influenza virus.

Aspirin (ASA) should never be given to children with the flu.

If anyone has the flu, they should avoid contact with those who are most at risk for developing influenza-related complications—seniors, young children, and people with chronic underlying medical conditions.

## Prevention Is Best

Up until about ten years ago, only children with chronic medical conditions including asthma, heart problems, and weakened immune systems such as happens with AIDS were thought to be at risk for flu-related complications. Tragically, during the 2003-04 season, there were several deaths in North America among otherwise healthy young children as a result of the flu. It seems that the flu is even more dangerous for normally healthy young children, too. For this reason, Canadian national vaccination guidelines currently recommend that all healthy children between six months and five years of age (six months to eight years of age in the US) receive an annual flu vaccine. Please check with your healthcare provider for specific details and updates. If you live outside Canada and the US, please check with your specific country's recommendations. The main point is that young and otherwise healthy children need to be vaccinated. In fact I feel that everyone should be getting the flu shot, as the more people vaccinated, the less the virus has a chance to spread in the community.

## Other Preventative Measures

Aside from the flu vaccine, here are some other steps that parents, schools, and others can take to help prevent the spread of the flu virus:

- Avoid close contact with people who are sick.
- Keep your child at home, if he or she is sick.
- Teach your children to cover their mouth and nose with a tissue when coughing or sneezing.
- Teach your children to wash their hands, especially before and after meals .

# Insect Bite Reactions

Insect bite reactions are common in young children. Children who have asthma or other allergies tend to have more exaggerated reactions to bites from insects such as mosquitoes, flies, and fleas.

Fortunately, most insect bite reactions are local rather than generalized, and although they may seem large and uncomfortable, the reassuring feature is that the reaction is indeed local. Although in most cases it is easy to distinguish a local reaction from anaphylaxis, if there is a doubt, do not hesitate to consult a healthcare provider. Most insect bite reactions can be treated quite simply by applying calamine lotion to the area. Giving antihistamines prior to exposure to insects does not appear to prevent reactions to bites. Insect bite reactions usually go away within one to three days. If the reaction persists beyond this or if it gets redder or more swollen (with or without pus), these may be signs of an infected reaction that may need to be treated with antibiotics.

## Insect Bite Prevention

Certainly the best way to prevent a reaction is to try to prevent the insect bite in the first place through the following measures:

- Avoid the use of scented soaps, perfumes, and hair sprays.
- Do not dress children in clothing with bright prints.
- Dress children in long pants and lightweight, long-sleeved shirts, socks, and shoes when going into an area with a lot of insects.
- Avoid areas where insects are found, such as garbage cans, pools of water, and even puddles.
- Use insect repellents containing DEET.

For more details, see Mosquito Bite Protection in the chapter on Keeping Baby Safe Outside the Home.

## When Are Insect Bite Reactions Dangerous?

Although much less common than a local reaction, symptoms of a generalized (anaphylactic) reaction to an insect bite extend beyond the area of the bite itself and include the following symptoms:

- Sudden difficulty breathing;
- Weakness or fainting;
- Itchy rash (hives) all over the body, not just around the bite location itself;
- Swelling of the face, including on the lip or tongue area.

Anaphylactic reactions usually occur following bee, wasp, or hornet stings. If a child ever experiences such a reaction, medical attention should be sought immediately, as unfortunately this can be fatal. Children who have had a sting-induced generalized (anaphylactic) reaction should have allergy tests to determine which venomous insect they are allergic to. Only children who are allergic to a stinging insect are prone to developing an anaphylactic reaction. Also, children who have had an anaphylactic reaction to a sting will need to carry an auto injector containing adrenalin (an EpiPen® or AllerjetTM ) to be administered in the case of a sting. Note that once the EpiPen® or similar auto injector is used, its effect will only last about thirty minutes. So if you live farther than thirty minutes away from your nearest hospital, you will need more than one EpiPen® on hand. Your allergist will provide you with specific details relevant to your situation.

The good news is that there are specific allergy shots for bee, wasp, and hornet sting allergies, which have been shown to be very effective in actually curing or getting rid of the allergy.

Note that insect repellents do not prevent stings from bees, wasps, or hornets.

# Lactose Intolerance

Lactose intolerance differs from cow's milk protein allergy. In order to understand the difference, one must know exactly what makes up cow's milk. Cow's milk straight from the cow contains several basic components: protein, sugar (specifically lactose), fat, vitamins, and nutrients such as the mineral calcium. When we talk about cow's milk allergy, which is the most common food allergy in children, we mean that a child is actually allergic to the protein in cow's milk. In other words, the child's body reacts to the cow's milk protein, producing symptoms that can range from a rash, difficulty breathing, and swelling of the face and mouth area, to excessive crying, vomiting, and diarrhea.

## What Is Lactose Intolerance?

Lactose intolerance is the intestine's inability to digest the milk sugar known as lactose; lactose in milk cannot be absorbed by the body. But ordinarily, everyone has an enzyme in their digestive system called lactase that breaks down lactose into smaller parts that the intestine can absorb. In cases of lactose intolerance, the lactase enzyme is either absent or reduced, leaving the person unable to break down the lactose properly in order to digest it. The lactose then remains in the intestine, causing the typical symptoms of lactose intolerance, which include excess gas, bloating, abdominal pain, and diarrhea. Permanent lactose intolerance rarely occurs in children, but as they get older it can develop, and in some ethnic groups, the rate of lactose intolerance in adults is quite high. Temporary or transient lactose intolerance can occur in children, often after a bout of gastroenteritis that causes a temporary decrease in intestinal lactase, but this usually resolves within a few weeks.

Lactose intolerance is not dangerous, but it can cause discomfort. The treatment is simply to avoid lactose in milk, which is easily achieved by using lactose-free cow's milk and taking pills such as Lactaid® or Lactease® before eating lactose-containing foods like ice cream. In this situation, cow's milk protein is not a problem and, therefore, need not be avoided.

# Lyme Disease

Lyme disease is caused by a bacterium called Borrelia. Humans are exposed to this germ by getting bitten by the blacklegged tick, also known as a deer tick. Ticks come in contact with the bacteria and get infected when they feed on infected animals; they can then pass it to humans by biting them. Although most cases initially occur in New England and the Eastern/mid-Atlantic states in the US, Lyme disease has also been reported in Canada.

Lyme disease occurs in both adults and children. Symptoms usually begin within a few weeks after the tick bite and include these symptoms:

- Fever;
- Fatigue;
- Headache;
- Muscle and joint pain;
- Skin rash with the specific look of a bull's-eye.

## Confirming and Treating Lyme Disease

Confirming the diagnosis of Lyme disease requires special blood tests. Once the diagnosis is made, the treatment is antibiotics for up to twenty-eight days, either by mouth or intravenously, depending on the individual situation. Fortunately with prompt antibiotic treatment, the infection usually goes away without any complications or problems.

Left untreated, the disease can cause more serious problems such as arthritis, facial paralysis (an inability to move the face muscles), meningitis, and heart infection (also known as carditis). These complications usually occur when the disease is not detected and treated early.

## Preventing Lyme Disease

Needless to say, preventing Lyme disease is better than getting it. So I want to talk a bit about ticks and how to avoid getting tick bites. Ticks are small insects about the size of a sesame seed, but when they feed off human blood, they grow much larger, to about three-quarters of an inch. Ticks do not fly, but move slowly on the ground and they may settle on tall grass. Also, it is important to know that a bite from a tick does not always cause Lyme disease.

If you live or work near woods or overgrown bush, if you hike, camp, fish, or hunt, or if you have an outdoor job working in landscaping and brush areas, you have a higher chance of getting Lyme disease, especially in areas where the infection is known to be found.

Here are some tips for avoiding ticks:

- Wear light coloured clothing, with long pants and a long-sleeved shirt.
- Wear closed shoes and socks, and tuck your pants into your socks. Do not wear sandals.
- Use a tick repellent containing DEET.
- Keep your grass well cut.
- Put a tick and flea collar on your pet.

If you are in a region where you know there are ticks, make sure you check yourself and your children for ticks, especially in the groin, scalp, and armpit areas. Taking a shower upon returning from a grassy or wooded area is also helpful in removing ticks.

If you do find a tick on your skin or your child's skin, remove it with a pair of tweezers as soon as possible, and wash and disinfect your hands as well as the bite area. If the tick has been there for more than twenty-four hours, or if you have any other concerns, please contact your healthcare provider.

# Lymph Nodes

Lymph nodes are responsible for protecting the body against infection, and like all lymph tissue including tonsils and adenoids, they tend to increase in size during childhood and then shrink and as a child reaches adolescence.

## Where Are Lymph Nodes Found?

The most common area where we see lymph nodes is the neck area—usually the region under the jaw and sometimes in the back of the neck. Lymph nodes can also be felt or noticed, especially in babies, at the area of the back of the head called the occipital area and, at times, right behind the ears. Lymph nodes can also be found in the groin and armpit areas.

## What Causes Lymph Nodes To Enlarge?

Most lymph nodes feel like small peas, but they can get bigger, usually as a reaction to a nearby infection. For example, a child with a throat infection will usually have enlarged nodes in the neck area. A child with a skin infection around the thigh may have enlarged nodes on the same side in the groin (also known as the inguinal area). This enlargement means that the lymph nodes have reacted to a local infection to help fend it off. As a reflection of a local infection, nodes get bigger, then shrink as the infection clears. This cycle can continue a few times during childhood.

## Can Enlarged Lymph Nodes Be a Serious Problem?

In general, healthcare providers can tell by feeling them whether the nodes are following a normal pattern, based on their size, texture, and location.

A possible yet infrequent complication of an enlarged lymph node is a bacterial infection of the node itself, known as adenitis. In this case, one can easily tell that there is an infection as the node becomes very big, tender, painful, and is quite red. In some cases, there may even be associated fever. How are these treated? When the infection is small and detected early enough, antibiotics taken by mouth are usually prescribed. In other cases, the child may need to be admitted to hospital for intravenous antibiotics and possibly to drain the infected node, which usually contains pus.

## When to Take Action

Of course, not all bumps are nodes, and while most visible or noticeable nodes are not troublesome, in rare cases, the cause may be more serious, such as cancer (lymphoma). This is why lymph nodes persisting in an enlarged form or getting bigger beyond a six-week period are usually removed in a biopsy and examined microscopically. Happily, this is quite unusual; most noticeable lymph nodes in children are not serious and shrink or go away on their own.

# Measles

Many people are surprised to discover that measles is a common cause of death in children worldwide today. Yes, I said, "Today," in the 21st century. In developing areas like Sub-Saharan Africa, measles is among the top causes of death in the millions of children who tragically die every year. Thanks to vaccinations and better nutrition, measles is now very rare in North America and other developed areas of the world.

## What Causes Measles?

Measles, also known as rubeola or red measles, is caused by the measles virus. This virus is highly contagious and is spread by droplet or direct contact with droplets from the nose, mouth, and throat of an infected person or with articles that have come into contact with nasal or throat secretions. This is similar to how the influenza virus spreads.

## Measles Symptoms

The incubation period or the time between contact and appearance of first symptoms is between eight and twelve days. The initial symptoms of measles include runny nose, red eyes, and fever. Three to four days later, a red rash develops on the face and spreads to the rest of the body. The rash is not usually itchy, and lasts from four to seven days. People with measles are contagious for four days before the onset of the rash up to four days after the appearance of the rash. Serious complications include severe lung and brain infections. Those most susceptible to complications and death include malnourished young children and persons with underlying immune weakness. The death rate of measles is between one and three per thousand persons infected. So this is a very serious and potentially deadly infection.

## How Is Measles Confirmed?

The diagnosis is suspected by a physician who on physical examination may see white spots inside the mouth called Koplik spots. However, the definite diagnosis can only be made by either a blood test, urine test, or nasal swab.

## Measles Prevention

There is no specific treatment for measles. So this is why prevention through vaccination is the best option. One dose of measles vaccine provides 85 percent to 95 percent immunity and a second booster dose increases that rate to as high as 99 percent. The first dose is usually given after the first birthday and a booster shot is administered at eighteen months of age. Anyone diagnosed with measles should be excluded from school, childcare facilities, and work until four days after the appearance of the rash. Most of the North American population is protected, either directly from the vaccination, or indirectly because so many people have been vaccinated. The greater the number of people who have been vaccinated, the less the virus has a chance to circulate among us. This is called herd immunity. Despite this, there have been recent measles outbreaks across North America. Most cases are in individuals who have brought the infection from other countries or in those not vaccinated or only partially vaccinated.

# Meningitis

The term "meningitis" means an infection of the covering of the brain, which is known as the meninges. Although there are multiple causes, the two major germ categories are bacterial and viral. Viral meningitis, which occurs mostly during the summer months, goes away on its own, and usually causes no significant complications. In this chapter, I will discuss bacterial meningitis in children. The spread of these bacteria from person to person is airborne through respiratory droplets.

## What Are the Causes of Bacterial Meningitis?

In children over three months, there are three main bacteria that cause meningitis:

*Streptococcus pneumoniae* (the most common);
*Hemophilus influenzae*;
*Neisseria meningitidis* (also known as meningococcus).

The first two bacteria, *Streptococcus pneumoniae* and *Hemophilus influenzae*, are also the main bacterial causes of ear and other respiratory infections, including pneumonia and sinusitis. Meningococcus has been the cause of the recent outbreaks of bacterial meningitis. This particular infection is discussed later in greater detail.

## Symptoms of Meningitis

In general, children with meningitis look very ill and the specific signs and symptoms vary with age. In older children, the symptoms may include:

- Fever;
- Stiff neck;
- Headache;
- Vomiting.

In younger children, especially babies less than three months, the symptoms are very nonspecific. For example, irritability, poor feeding, increased sleepiness with and even without a fever. Therefore, it is usually difficult to determine just by symptoms whether a baby has meningitis or not. When examining an older child, the healthcare provider can look for signs of meningitis by bending the neck, which is usually stiff. Also, by bending the neck forward, the hips move upwards in persons with meningitis. These are specific signs of meningitis in older children and adults, which are usually absent in babies.

## How Is Meningitis Confirmed?

In children with suspected meningitis, the only way the diagnosis can be definitively confirmed is by a procedure called a lumbar puncture (also known as a spinal tap). This relatively safe procedure involves placing a hollow needle between the spinal bones in the middle of the lower back after the area has been frozen. Spinal fluid is then collected into small test tubes and sent for analysis. A positive spinal tap means that a child has meningitis, and the liquid will then be tested to see which bacteria—if any—are the cause. If no bacteria are found, but the spinal fluid is abnormal, the liquid may be tested for viruses or other causes.

## Consequences of Bacterial Meningitis

Bacterial meningitis is an extremely dangerous infection. The associated problems and complications range from brain-related infections and damage (such as deafness, paralysis, seizures, and even mental retardation), to the spread of infection through the blood, even tragically to death.

## Meningitis Treatment

Bacterial meningitis is treated with intravenous antibiotics, which fortunately have been able to decrease and/or prevent the associated potential complications. However, despite antibiotic use, the death rate from bacterial meningitis is about 10 percent.

## What if a Child Comes Into Contact With a Person who Develops Meningitis?

The answer depends on which bacteria are causing the meningitis. If the meningitis is caused by *Hemophilus influenzae* or *meningococcus*, preventative antibiotics (usually rifampin) taken by mouth are given to close contacts (household, barracks, dorm, school, and daycare). In the case of outbreaks or mini-epidemics of *meningococcus*, which occurred in the early 1990s and more during the winter season of 2000-01, and more recently in 2014, mass vaccination programs may be recommended by public health authorities.

## Is There a Single Meningitis Vaccine?

No. Because there are several bacteria that cause meningitis, there is no single meningitis vaccine protecting against all the possible bacterial causes. However, what has had a big impact on decreasing meningitis is the introduction of the *Hemophilus influenzae* vaccine, which is now given routinely to all children from two month of age. Hemophilus meningitis and other related infections have decreased significantly since the vaccination has been given universally. Unfortunately, this vaccination does not protect children from the other two bacteria, for which there are now separate vaccines available. The *Streptococcus pneumoniae* vaccine has been recommended for all children as part of their routine immunization, protecting them from this dangerous bacteria. In addition, there are also vaccines available to prevent meningococcal infections that are due to the various types of *Neisseria meningitidis* bacteria.

## Meningococcal Infection and Prevention

*Meningococcus* is the bacteria that has caused meningitis outbreaks across North America over the last two decades. Understandably, the presence of a meningitis epidemic in a community is very scary. There are several types of the meningococcus bacteria that cause infection in humans: A, B, C, Y, and W. Type B strains account for most of the recent *meningococcal* outbreaks.

## Why Is Meningococcal Infection so Dangerous?

This particular bacteria is quite dangerous because, in addition, to causing meningitis, it can enter the blood stream (called meningococcemia) and cause the body to go into shock, resulting in kidney failure and, unfortunately, possibly death. Tragically, the risk of dying from meningococcemia is about 17 percent. Therefore, not only can meningococcal infection result in meningitis, which in itself is bad enough, but it can also cause significant damage to the rest of the body. One of the difficulties with treating meningococcemia is that it can spread so quickly and cause such an overwhelming infection that even antibiotics and other supportive treatments cannot always stop the infection, explaining why the mortality rate is so high.

## How Is Meningococcus Spread?

The spread of *meningococcus* is usually from direct person-to-person contact through respiratory secretions. This is why outbreaks of infection occur more frequently in crowded conditions such as in the army, schools, and dormitories. People most prone to getting the infection from someone already infected are those who have had close prolonged contact. More than 50 percent of infections occur in children younger than five years old. There is also a higher incidence of this infection in fifteen to twenty-four year olds. The infections most frequently occur during the winter and spring months.

## Symptoms of Meningococcal Infection

If the child only gets meningitis, then the signs and symptoms are as described above for meningitis (see Symptoms of Meningitis). However, if the infection spreads into the blood, one of the main signs specific to meningococcemia is the development of little blue spots on the skin called petechiae, which grow rapidly and spread all over the body, eventually looking like large bruises. If a child ever develops such a rash, especially in the context of an outbreak of a meningococcal infection, medical attention should be sought immediately. Not all petechiae are due to meningococcemia, but this should be ruled out immediately, because if meningococcemia is either suspected or confirmed, immediate treatment and monitoring are essential.

## How Is Meningococcal Infection Treated?

People with full-blown meningococcemia are very ill because of this potentially deadly infection. Therefore, they require intensive medical therapy, support, and monitoring in addition to intravenous antibiotics.

## What Happens to Contacts of a Person With Meningococcal Infection?

The most important thing to do is treat the close contacts with antibiotics taken by mouth. When given promptly, preventative antibiotics have been shown to prevent infection very effectively.

## Vaccination Against Meningococcus

Effective vaccines preventing infections from several types of meningococcus—A, C, Y, and W—have been available for a few years. There are several vaccines, some protecting against C, and others against all four types. Very recently (2013), a new vaccine against Type B meningococcus was approved in several countries including Canada and the UK. Depending on where you are, the meningococcal vaccines may be given to children at school or available at your local clinic. Please speak to your healthcare provider or local public health agency to determine what vaccines are available and at what age.

If there is a meningococcal outbreak in your area, local public health authorities may recommend mass vaccination as this has been shown to be able to stop outbreaks. It must be noted that it takes several weeks for the vaccination to protect a person and, therefore, household contacts or those who have been in close contact with people with active meningococcal infection should receive antibiotics preventatively, even if they have been vaccinated as part of a public health campaign.

## What Else Can Parents Do to Protect Their Children?

The main thing that parents can do is be on the lookout for any petechiae or other signs of meningitis described above, especially under conditions of a local or community outbreak of infection. If parents are not sure, they should not take a chance, but seek medical attention just to be on the safe side.

# Mono

The actual medical term is infectious mononucleosis, and it is caused by the Epstein-Barr virus (EBV). Though most people in North America associate mono with teens and adults, it can infect children of all ages; in fact, in developing countries the average age of infection is two to four years of age.

## Symptoms of Mono

The symptoms and signs of mono are quite specific, but in younger children it can look like a cold. Often, we do not make an immediate diagnosis, because the symptoms mimic those of other viral infections.

The typical symptoms of mono include a period of a week or two of fever, feeling tired, and a very sore throat. Other typical signs of mono are enlarged glands in the neck region, a rash all over the body, and, less frequently, swelling around the eyes. When we examine children with possible mono, we find a tired-looking child, with very large (often whitish) tonsils, and swollen glands around the neck. Up to 50 percent of children with mono will develop an enlarged spleen. The diagnosis is confirmed by a specific blood test.

One of the most common complications of mono is not being able to swallow due to the very sore throat. Obviously, we recommend drinking as much fluid as possible, but avoiding fruit juices as these may hurt the already sore throat. As a matter of fact, milk shakes are a great idea in children with very sore throats. In extreme cases, when children cannot drink enough, they may become dehydrated and require hospitalization so they can receive fluids intravenously.

## How Long Can Mono Last?

The symptoms of mono typically persist for a two-to-three-week period and the fatigue can linger for up to one or two months.

## What Is the Treatment of Mono?

There is no specific treatment for mono as long as the child is drinking adequately. Young adults or adolescents with mono are typically very tired and will need to rest in bed. Usually, they will have little energy to do much else. As time goes by, they become more energetic and can return to normal activities, depending on how they feel. One important point to keep in mind is that an enlarged spleen can be easily damaged during physical activity. This is important, because a ruptured spleen can be fatal. For this reason, children with a mono-related enlarged spleen should not partake in any exercise or physical activity, especially a contact sport, even if they're feeling better.

When the child is feeling better, he or she should be reassessed by a healthcare provider. If the spleen size has returned to normal, physical exercise and activity can resume.

## The Kissing Disease

Mono is spread through the saliva. This is why it is known as the Kissing Disease. However, most commonly, it spreads by close contact or sharing kitchen and other utensils with an infected individual.

## Mumps

Mumps, also known as epidemic parotitis, is caused by the *Paramyxovirus*. This is an infection of the salivary (parotid) glands found in the neck region behind the lower jaw and below the ear. The virus infects these glands and causes them to swell. The virus is spread through respiratory droplets. A person with mumps is contagious during the period between one day before the swelling begins and three days after the swelling goes away.

The incubation period for mumps (the time between exposure and symptoms starting) is usually between fourteen and twenty-four days. The symptoms begin with pain in the neck area and then the swelling becomes obvious, either on one or both sides of the neck. There can be some low to moderate fever, and the swelling goes away within a week or so. The diagnosis is made by a throat swab, a urine sample, and/or blood tests.

There is no specific treatment for mumps and most cases resolve without a problem. However, there are some rare, yet potentially serious complications of mumps, including meningitis and, in older boys, infection of the testicles (orchitis), which can lead to future infertility.

The best approach is ensuring that your child is fully immunized against mumps. The mumps vaccine is part of the routine childhood vaccine series. Thanks to the vaccine, mumps cases are now relatively rare.

# Nosebleeds

Nosebleeds, also known as "Epistaxis," are common in children and fortunately not usually associated with any serious underlying problem. Most of the time, nosebleeds stop on their own without any specific treatment. With age the tendency for nosebleeds decreases.

## What Causes Nosebleeds?

An obvious cause is nasal trauma or injury, including picking the nose. We also know, that the tendency to have nosebleeds increases during the winter months when the dry air irritates the inside lining of the nose resulting in bleeding. Interestingly, there seems to be a family tendency. In other words, children with recurring nosebleeds often have relatives who have had the same. We also know that children with large adenoids, nasal allergies, and chronic sinusitis tend to have more nosebleeds. In very rare circumstances, frequent or excessive nosebleeds may reflect a bleeding problem such as low platelet counts or a lack of certain blood clotting factors (i.e. hemophilia). In these cases there is a generalized bleeding tendency (cuts tend to bleed more than normal, etcetera), making it relatively easy to distinguish a normal child from one who has a blood clotting problem. Again, let me reiterate, most children with epistaxis are otherwise normal.

## Treating Nosebleeds

There are two aspects to treatment: trying to stop a nosebleed and trying to prevent it. While most nosebleeds stop on their own within a few minutes, compressing or clamping the nose between the thumb and index finger will help. Contrary to what most people do, the head should be tilted forwards and not backwards. Tilting the head backwards will cause the blood to trickle down the child's throat, possibly resulting in coughing, choking, or swallowing the blood. In most children, gentle nose compression or pressure will stop the bleeding easily. If the bleeding persists, medical attention should be sought as application of certain medications and/or the insertion of nasal packing (cotton) gauzes will likely be needed. Certain children with recurrent nosebleeds may need an evaluation by an ENT doctor who will look for any bleeding site (a weakened blood vessel) and burn or cauterize it with silver nitrate application.

## Preventing Nosebleeds

Prevention of nosebleeds is the other aspect of treatment. Obviously, avoidance of trauma and wearing appropriate face protection during sports is important. Also, you should try to teach your kids not to pick their nose. During the winter months, make sure that the humidity in the house is adequate (about 40 percent). A humidifier can be used to bring the humidity up to this normal level. Another approach is to apply petroleum gel (Vaseline®) or nasal saline lubricating gel inside the nostrils at night. By keeping the inside lining of the nose moist, this treatment can also help prevent nosebleeds.

# Pneumonia

Pneumonia means an infection of the lungs. In the early 1900s, pneumonia was responsible for many deaths, even in children. Fortunately, with the invention of antibiotics and certain vaccines, the occurrence of pneumonia is less common today and can be effectively treated in most cases.

## What Causes Pneumonia?

There are several types of germs that can cause an infection of the lungs: bacterial and viral. Although there are many different types of bacteria and viruses that can cause pneumonia, they tend to be related to age and other circumstances. For example, the bacteria that cause pneumonia in newborns differ from those that cause the same infection in older children. Similarly, seemingly harmless germs may cause pneumonia in persons with weakened immune or defence systems. These same germs would, however, cause no problem in persons who are healthy.

## Symptoms of Pneumonia

The symptoms of pneumonia in children depend on the age. In younger children, it may be just fever or irritability. At any age, there can be the nonspecific symptoms such as irritability and decreased appetite or feeding, without any specific respiratory or chest symptoms. In newborns, a specific type of pneumonia (Group B Streptococcus) can present soon after birth with difficulty breathing. As children get older, the symptoms of pneumonia become more specific:

- Cough;
- Fever;
- Difficulty breathing.

**Important point:** In some children, a persistent high fever (for more than four days) can be the only sign of pneumonia.

## How Is Pneumonia Confirmed?

Although the healthcare provider can sometimes hear specific chest noises with a stethoscope that suggest pneumonia, the diagnosis is absolutely confirmed by a chest X-ray. As a matter of fact, in young children, the chest X-ray can be abnormal, even if the chest examination is normal.

## How Is Pneumonia Treated?

For viral pneumonia, there is no treatment, although in most cases the healthcare provider cannot tell if the cause is viral and will treat all pneumonias with antibiotics. Which antibiotic and how it is administered depend on the age and overall condition of the child. In general, children less than three months of age with pneumonia are admitted to hospital for intravenous antibiotics, oxygen treatment, and rehydration, as they tend to be dehydrated. Of course, children with weakened immune systems are usually hospitalized and may need different (stronger) antibiotics than the children with normal immune systems.

In older children who are otherwise well, are drinking well, and do not need oxygen, antibiotics taken by mouth that can be given at home are prescribed. During the first forty-eight hours of antibiotics, the child is still considered contagious and still may have fever. In this case, acetaminophen can be given for the fever as needed, according to the age and weight of the child. If after forty-eight hours of antibiotics, the child still has a fever or is not getting better, the child should be re-examined by a healthcare provider.

After the full antibiotic treatment course, children usually fully recover and there is no need to repeat the chest X-ray in typical non-complicated cases. However, if the child was very ill, or had a large or severe pneumonia, a repeat chest X-ray may be recommended to make sure the pneumonia has cleared. If this is the case, a repeat X-ray is performed six to eight weeks later.

## Recurrent Pneumonia

Fortunately, most children recover fully and do not have repeated episodes of pneumonia. However, if a child has recurrent pneumonia, this may be a sign of an underlying medical problem including a weakened immune system, foreign body aspiration (having aspirated or choked on something that lodges in the lungs or bronchial tubes), or a structural defect of the lungs or bronchi. Obviously in such situations, both the treatment and follow-up approach would be different than for the typical pneumonia in a normal child. Specific tests including blood tests, sweat chloride (a test for cystic fibrosis), CT scans, and other investigations may be necessary.

# Pyloric Stenosis

Pyloric Stenosis is a condition that usually occurs in firstborn baby boys, between the ages of three to six weeks. The main symptom of pyloric stenosis is persistent and progressively worsening vomiting in an otherwise healthy baby.

## What Is the Cause of Pyloric Stenosis?

When food enters the stomach, the stomach muscles contract and churn the food for easier digestion. Normally, the food then passes through the stomach into the small intestine. At the end or outlet of the stomach leading into the small intestine is the pylorus, which is a muscular, elastic-like sphincter. In pyloric stenosis, for reasons not well understood, the pylorus is too big or hypertrophied. In other words, the pyloric muscle gets too thick and actually blocks the food from leaving the stomach. This results in persistent vomiting that continues to worsen unless the problem is treated.

## Symptoms of Pyloric Stenosis

Generally, babies with pyloric stenosis are initially otherwise well, without any fever, pain, or other symptoms. In fact, they are often quite hungry. The main symptom, which is highly suggestive of pyloric stenosis, is projectile vomiting. This means that vomit is ejected quite far from the baby with great force. The stomach is contracting and trying to push the food into the intestine, but the food is blocked by the enlarged pylorus, so it is pushed upwards instead.

## How Is Pyloric Stenosis Confirmed?

Usually the history of the projectile vomiting in a three- to six-week-old otherwise well baby boy raises high suspicions of pyloric stenosis.

On physical examination, the healthcare provider may find signs of dehydration, and may actually notice the baby's abdomen is distended or ballooned, because the stomach is stretched. Sometimes, the healthcare provider may actually feel the olive-like pylorus while examining the baby's belly. An X-ray and ultrasound will confirm the diagnosis. Blood tests will be taken to assess the degree of dehydration.

## How Is Pyloric Stenosis Treated ?

The only definitive treatment of pyloric stenosis is an operation called a pyloromyotomy. Before surgery, the baby is given fluids through an intravenous and is not allowed to feed. A tube may be inserted into the stomach through the nose to relieve the distension or bloated abdomen. During the operation, the surgeon cuts and removes the excess muscle of the pylorus, unblocking the stomach and thus resolving the problem. The operation lasts less than an hour and the baby usually recovers fully very quickly. The baby can usually start feeding six to eight hours after the operation.

Fortunately, almost all babies do very well after the operation and have no recurrence nor are there any long-term consequences.

# Roseola

Roseola is a childhood viral infection also known as exanthem subitum or sixth disease. Roseola is self-limiting, in other words, it goes away on its own. The roseola virus tends to cause infections in children younger than two years of age. This infection is rare in children less than three months or older than four years of age.

## Roseola Symptoms

Typically, roseola causes initially fever with a bit of irritability and no other obvious symptoms. The fever characteristically lasts for up to three to four days and then goes away on its own. At the same time, a rash (usually on the whole body) comes out. The roseola rash usually lasts another few days, but without fever. This is the distinguishing feature of roseola: the rash appears only after the fever breaks. This pattern in the history is very typical for roseola. There are, of course, other viruses that cause fever and rash, but none of them first presents with fever only and then a rash once the fever subsides. Most of the other viral infections feature rash and fever at the same time.

## How Is Roseola Spread?

The roseola virus is thought to spread, like many other viruses, through respiratory secretions. The incubation period (time between exposure to the virus and actually developing symptoms), is between five and fourteen days. Most cases of roseola occur during the spring, summer, and fall periods. Once a child gets roseola, this infection does not recur.

## Is There a Specific Treatment?

There is no specific treatment for roseola, except for fever medication (such as acetaminophen) as needed. Remember that aspirin (acetylsalicylic acid (ASA)) should never be used in children. Additionally, no special precautions or control measures are necessary for children or adults who have come into in contact with someone with roseola.

# Rubella (German Measles)

Rubella, sometimes known as German measles or three-day measles is caused by the T*ogaviridae virus*. Note that **German measles is not the same as measles**. Although, it is transmitted from one person to another by respiratory droplets, the rubella virus can also be passed through the blood from an infected mother to her baby during pregnancy. Referred to as congenital rubella, rubella contracted this way can cause significant and permanent damage to the baby, especially if the infection occurs early on during the pregnancy. This is why pregnant mothers and women planning to become pregnant are routinely tested for evidence of past rubella infection or vaccination. If a person has had either a rubella vaccination, or a rubella infection in the past, they are considered protected against this infection

After a fourteen to twenty-one day incubation period, rubella infections start with mild nonspecific, cold-like symptoms, with pain along the lymph nodes of the neck region and throat. After about twenty-four hours, a rash develops all over the body. The rash usually disappears within three days. People with rubella are contagious from one week before to one week after the rash appears. There is no available treatment and the infection usually resolves on its own without any consequences. Rare complications of rubella include arthritis, infection of the nerves (neuritis) and, in some extremely rare cases, chronic brain infections.

## Rubella Prevention

The best approach is ensuring that your child is immunized against rubella. The rubella vaccine is part of the routine childhood vaccine series. Thanks to the vaccine, rubella cases are now relatively rare. For women who plan to be pregnant and have not yet been vaccinated against rubella, or are unsure whether they have had rubella or a vaccine against the disease, it is a good idea to speak to your healthcare provider to ensure you are protected against rubella.

# Scarlet Fever

Scarlet fever is an infection of the throat or tonsils caused by the streptococcus bacterium, which is the same germ that causes strep throat. However, the scarlet fever bacterium also produces a toxin that causes other symptoms not usually seen with a strep throat. As with strep throat, this infection is seen mostly in school-age children and much less frequently in children less than three years of age. For more information on strep throat and tonsil infections please read the chapter on Tonsils and Tonsil Infections.

## Symptoms of Scarlet Fever

Children with scarlet fever look quite sick and have the following symptoms:

- Sore throat;
- High fever;
- Swollen neck glands;
- Headache and/or abdominal pain;
- A rash.

## The Scarlet Fever Rash

The symptoms described above can be seen in other types of infections as well. But the scarlet fever rash is what distinguishes this illness from others. The rash usually appears several days after the sore throat, starting on the child's neck and face, and spreading down to the chest and back. The rash makes the skin feel rough, just like sandpaper. The areas affected by the rash will turn white when you press on them. One feature very characteristic for the scarlet fever rash is that it is most concentrated around the armpit and groin areas.

## Scarlet Fever Confirmation

A healthcare provider usually can make the diagnosis by the characteristic rash and by looking in the child's throat. The tonsils and the back of the throat may be covered with a whitish coating or appear red and swollen. The tongue may have a white coating or have red spots (called a strawberry tongue). Also, the area around the mouth may be pale. The diagnosis is confirmed by obtaining a sample of the fluids from your child's throat with a cotton swab. This throat swab test will identify the *streptococcus* bacteria.

## Scarlet Fever Treatment

For confirmed scarlet fever infection, antibiotics will be prescribed. You should give the medicine on time and for as many days as directed. If you skip doses or stop the medicine too soon, the infection may return. It usually takes about twenty-four to forty-eight hours for the fever to fall and the child to start feeling better. In the meantime, make sure the child is drinking well and enough. Also during this time, acetaminophen can be given for fever. If your child worsens or the fever persists despite forty-eight hours of antibiotics contact your healthcare provider.

## Is Scarlet Fever Contagious?

Just like strep throat infections, scarlet fever is considered contagious. It spreads from one person to another through airborne respiratory droplets, mostly in crowded or close-contact areas such as schools and daycares. A child is considered to no longer be contagious after a full twenty-four hours of antibiotics.

## Is Scarlet Fever Dangerous?

As with strep throat, the infection of scarlet fever can spread into the ears, sinuses, and the area behind the tonsils. Other complications of untreated streptococcal throat infections can appear several weeks after the infection. These are referred to as non-infectious complications: kidney inflammation and heart damage (acute rheumatic fever). It is for these reasons that it is necessary to complete the whole prescribed course of the antibiotics, even if the child starts to feel better. Fortunately, with treatment most children recover fully without any complications.

# SIDS: Sudden Infant Death Syndrome

Tragically, SIDS, sometimes referred to as crib death, is a leading cause of death in babies. In the US, there are more than two thousand SIDS deaths per year. Ninety percent of SIDS deaths occur during the first six months of life, most between two and four months of age. The SIDS death rate has been steadily decreasing since the new recommendation was issued to place all babies on their backs to sleep. SIDS occurs more often in male babies. Also, African-American and Native American infants have a higher rate of SIDS as compared with Caucasian, Asian, and Hispanic babies.

It is also known that SIDS victims are more likely to be born to a young mother with a lower educational level. SIDS tends to occur more in colder geographic areas and during the winter. Recent illness, such as an upper respiratory infection or gastroenteritis, is commonly reported in relation to the baby's death.

## What Causes SIDS?

SIDS is technically defined as the sudden death of a previously healthy baby younger than one year of age. An infant's death is attributed to SIDS only if no other cause of that death is found after a thorough investigation. There are many misconceptions about what causes SIDS, and although the exact cause is not understood, it is known that SIDS is not caused by infections, vaccinations, or immunizations.

SIDS is not thought to be caused by suffocation, vomiting, choking, or child abuse. The current thinking seems to focus on three main factors: the age of the child, combined with a problem in the control of breathing, as well as the presence of certain risk factors. These risk factors include the following:

- Prone sleeping position (sleeping on the stomach);
- Soft bedding;
- Cigarette smoke exposure (even during pregnancy);
- Overheating;
- Prematurity.

**NOTE: Prone sleeping (sleeping on the stomach)**, the most important risk factor within a parent's control, increases the risk of SIDS by ten to fifteen times.

## Prevention of SIDS

The only and best approach to SIDS is prevention, aiming to eliminate some of the risks that are within a parent's control.

### Sleep Position

**Sleeping your baby on her back is the most effective way to reduce the risk of SIDS.** This applies to night-time as well as daytime naps at home, at the babysitter's, and even in daycare. SIDS can occur during the day and 20 percent of SIDS deaths occur in childcare settings, while a baby is at the babysitter's or at daycare. Remember that a baby can be in the prone position (on their stomach) while he is awake. Since experts began promoting the baby-on-back sleep position in 1992, the number of SIDS deaths in the US has declined by 40 percent from 1.2 to 0.7 deaths per thousand births.

**Important:** Babies who sleep on their side are at twice the risk of SIDS as babies who sleep on their backs. The side position is not very stable, so a baby can easily roll onto the prone (on stomach) position.

Here are some other tips on how to make sure your baby's sleep environment is safe:

- In baby's crib: Avoid soft bedding, including blankets, comforters, quilts, pillows, stuffed toys, sheepskins, and crib bumpers.
- If blankets are necessary, only one thin blanket should be used, and it should be tucked in so that it cannot cover baby's head. In cold weather, a blanket sleeper is an alternative to a blanket.
- Select a crib that conforms to current safety and consumer standards, which has a firm and snug-fitting mattress.
- Never put a baby to sleep on a waterbed, sofa, couch, soft mattress, pillow, adult bed, or other soft surface.
- Avoid overheating your baby. Use light clothes for sleep and keep the room at a temperature of about 20° C (70° F).
- It's important to realize that removing risk factors decreases but does not completely eliminate the risk of SIDS.

#### No Smoking

Cigarette smoke exposure during pregnancy and second-hand smoke exposure after birth are important risk factors for SIDS. The more a baby is exposed to smoke, the higher the risk. This is one risk factor that parents can definitely control.

#### Breastfeeding Protects Against SIDS

For reasons not well understood, breastfeeding may have a protective effect against SIDS. This is yet another good reason to breastfeed your baby.

## Practical Issues

### Are There Adverse Effects if Babies Sleep on Their Back all the Time?

Very few. Studies have shown that babies who sleep on their backs have a slightly higher incidence of diaper rash and cradle cap as compared with babies who sleep on their stomachs. A flattening of the back part of the baby's head (positional occipital plagiocephaly) tends to be more common in babies who sleep on their backs. See the chapter on Head, Neck, and Related Concerns in the previous section of this book.

### Can My Baby Choke When Sleeping on his Back?

Multiple studies have not shown any increase in the rate of choking (aspiration of spit-up) related to sleeping on the back.

### Can I Ever Put My Baby On His Stomach?

Yes. The baby-on-back position recommendation applies only for sleep time. As a matter of fact, the American Academy of Pediatrics recommends that infants spend time on their tummy every day while awake and supervised. This decreases the incidence of positional plagiocephaly and also promotes motor development.

### Is Sleeping With Baby Dangerous?

Co-sleeping (sharing a bed with your baby) on the surface seems to make breastfeeding easier and is more convenient for tired parents. Sleeping with baby in the same bed as the parents occurs in many cultures outside North America. However, there is much controversy about the benefits and risks of co-sleeping. The fear is that although co-sleeping may facilitate breastfeeding and promote bonding, it may also result in overheating, exposure to passive cigarette smoke, and the risk of smothering or suffocation, all factors known to be associated with SIDS.

For years, health experts have been warning parents that babies need to be put to bed in a safe sleep environment. Unsafe sleep environments include parents' beds. Babies can be accidentally smothered by a parent, and adult mattresses are not suited for babies. Experts also fear that baby may be sleeping on a soft mattress with pillows and quilts, and may be at risk of getting caught or trapped between the bed and the wall, or the bed and the headboard. According to the American Academy of Pediatrics, co-sleeping does not protect against SIDS and in fact, may increase the risk of accidental suffocation.

My recommendation is that parents can be close to their baby by placing the baby's crib next to their bed. In this way, they can respond to baby's needs immediately, including quick access to breastfeeding, while not putting the baby at risk. I do not think that this prevents effective breastfeeding or bonding with baby.

Our babies are among our most precious treasures in life. It is worth every effort to make sure that their home and sleep environments are as safe as possible!

## Sinuses and Sinus Infections

The sinuses are the hollow cavities in the facial bones. There are several sinuses including below the eyes (maxillary), above the eyes (frontal), and behind the nose (ethmoid). Sinuses are part the respiratory tract, covered with respiratory mucosa or lining just as the lungs and bronchi are.

Babies are born with fewer sinuses, only with the maxillary and ethmoid sinuses. As they get older, their frontal sinuses develop, and the ethmoid and maxillary sinuses continue to grow.

### What is Sinusitis?

Sinusitis is an infection, either viral or bacterial, of the sinuses. The exact same bacteria that cause ear infections cause sinusitis. Normally, fluid in the sinuses drains into the nose. When these are blocked and not working properly, the fluid backs up and becomes infected by the bacteria. The typical symptoms of a sinus infection are usually pain around the sinus, pain around the eye, and green discharge coming out of the nose. In younger children, the symptoms are less specific, including irritability, prolonged fever, or a cold that won't go away. Importantly they may cough a lot, especially when they lie down at night. X-rays or CT scans are the only way to confirm the presence of a sinus infection or problem.

There are three types of sinusitis, depending on how long the infection has been going on:

- Acute sinusitis: symptoms have lasted less than two weeks.
- Sub-acute sinusitis: symptoms last for up to two months.
- Chronic sinusitis: symptoms recur or are persistent for more than two months.

## Treatment of Sinusitis

Antibiotics taken by mouth are usually required to treat sinusitis. The duration and type of antibiotic depends on the age of the child, the individual situation, and the duration of symptoms. One potentially serious complication of sinus infections in children is periorbital cellulitis. This is when the bacteria that cause the sinus infection spread to the area around the eye. This relatively rare condition requires admission to hospital for intravenous antibiotics and evaluation by an eye specialist (ophthalmologist).

# Swimmer's Ear

Both adults and children can develop swimmer's ear, especially during the summer months. Also known as otitis, swimmer's ear is commonly confused with the typical ear infections we see in children. However, these two types of conditions differ with respect not only to the cause and symptoms, but also to the treatments.

The term "otitis" means inflammation or infection of the ear and "externa" means outer or external. Thus, the term "otitis externa" refers to an infection or irritation of the outer ear canal caused by bacteria or fungi that are commonly found in lakes and oceans. Otitis externa tends to occur less frequently after swimming in pool water, because of the chlorine, which technically renders the water sterile. However, if the pool is not well chlorinated, swimmer's ear can occur after swimming in pools, too.

Swimmer's ear causes the following symptoms:

- Pain (especially in the ear canal);
- Itchiness of the ear;
- Oozing of pus or liquid from the affected ear;
- Pain worsens when moving the ear itself.

One of the differences between this type of infection and otitis media, the typical ear infection that we hear about in children, is that otitis externa does not affect the eardrum or the area behind it, known as the middle ear space. By examining the ear through an otoscope, a healthcare provider can usually easily distinguish swimmer's ear from otitis media. In swimmer's ear, the outer ear canal is red and irritated, whereas in otitis media, it is the eardrum itself that is red and infected. In contrast, this is not the case in swimmer's ear. Because it tends to occur during the swimming season, swimmer's ear is seen more frequently in the summer; otitis media, on the other hand, tends to occur more during the winter months.

## How Is Swimmer's Ear Treated ?

Again, the approach is not the same as for a middle ear infection, which is treated by antibiotics taken by mouth. For swimmer's ear, antibiotic/anti-inflammatory drops are prescribed and placed directly into the ear. The treatment is usually for five to seven days, and the symptoms improve within a day or two after starting the drops. Swimmer's ear very rarely causes any other more serious complications or problems.

## Swimmer's Ear Can Be Prevented

- By wearing a bathing cap that covers the ear canal while swimming for prolonged periods in a lake or at the beach;
- By drying out the ear canal after swimming. Gently passing a hair dryer over the ear may help; and
- By not swimming in pools that appear dirty or that are not properly chlorinated.

# Thrush

Oral thrush is a yeast infection that affects the mouth. It causes creamy white patches to form on the tongue or inner cheeks. These patches can be painful, but in many cases, the only signs are the white spots on the tongue or inner cheek areas of the mouth. Babies with thrush may have trouble feeding. Thrush is seldom serious in healthy children. Thrush is common in infants and toddlers. Babies sometimes pass the infection to their mothers. In most cases, thrush isn't a medical emergency. Call your healthcare provider if your baby develops symptoms of thrush.

## Treating Thrush

Babies with thrush are treated with a liquid antifungal medication. The liquid is administered by a dropper to be applied and spread directly on the affected area of the tongue and mouth, with a Q-tip®. The baby should not swallow the liquid medicine; there is no danger to your baby if she swallows the medicine, but it will not work unless it is rubbed onto the affected areas. Also, if your baby uses a pacifier, make sure you sterilize the pacifier each time you apply the medicine to prevent reinfection.

# Tonsils and Tonsil Infections

The tonsils are two little bumps or nodes found in the back of the throat at the end of the tongue. Tonsils are thought to be related to the development of the immune system and are part of the lymphatic tissue. Although older children and adults can live without them, tonsils are probably more important for the development of our immune system during pregnancy, before we are born.

The tonsils are small at birth and during infancy. Between the ages of five and ten, they start to get bigger on their own. Eventually after the age of twelve they start to shrink on their own. In the meantime, they can get infected and enlarge enough to cause problems. Some children's tonsils get so big that they are unable to breathe properly, especially at night. In addition, enlarged tonsils can also prevent a child from eating or swallowing well. Most tonsil-related problems occur in children over the age of two years, but can, less commonly, be seen in younger children too.

## Tonsillitis

Tonsillitis is an infection of the tonsils caused either by viruses or by bacteria. The usual bacteria causing tonsil infections is *Streptococcus* also known as Strep throat. The symptoms of a tonsil infection include:

- Sore throat;
- Difficulty swallowing;
- Drooling;
- Not being able to fully open his or her mouth;
- Pain in the lymph nodes in the neck;
- Neck pain.

Sometimes there can be associated nonspecific symptoms of a throat or tonsil infection in young children including fever, headache, and even abdominal pain.

## Tonsillitis Treatment

Most throat or tonsil infections are caused by viruses and do not need any treatment. Usually with viral infections of the tonsils, there are other associated symptoms of a cold such as a runny nose and cough. Strep throat, on the other hand, usually causes a very sharp pain, in the throat without any other symptoms.

By examining the throat, a healthcare provider cannot tell whether it is a viral infection or a Strep throat. It is important to know the cause, because unlike viral infections, the streptococcal throat infections can cause complications such as local spread to the back of the throat and longer term kidney and heart problems. Antibiotics given promptly will prevent most of these complications. To test for the presence of *Streptococcus*, a swab is taken from the back of the throat. If the test shows it is a Streptococcal infection, then antibiotics, usually taken by mouth, are prescribed. You should give the medicine on time and for as many days as directed. It usually takes about twenty-four to forty-eight hours for the fever to fall and the child to start feeling better. In the meantime, make sure the child is drinking well and enough. Also during this time, acetaminophen can be given for fever. If your child worsens or the fever persists despite forty-eight hours of antibiotics contact your healthcare provider.

Note that very rarely the infection spreads into the throat to cause an abscess full of pus. This complication requires hospitalization for surgery to drain the pus as well as antibiotics given intravenously.

## Removing Tonsils

In most children, the tonsils will not cause any significant problems and therefore do not need to be surgically removed. However, in some situations they need to be removed surgically under general anesthesia. This operation is known as a tonsillectomy. Currently the indications for removing tonsils are:

- Recurrent (Strep) infections; more than six in a year.
- The tonsils are so enlarged that they block breathing and or preventing eating.
- The development of an abscess around the tonsils.

Note that children and adults can still get throat infections even if they have had their tonsils removed in the past. The throat infection in this circumstance is known as pharyngitis.

# Urinary Tract Infections

Urinary tract infections (UTIs) do occur in children and even in babies. The cause of a urinary tract infection is bacteria in the urine and bladder. The bacteria can potentially infect the kidney and even enter the blood. In babies, the immune system is not as strong as in older children, so the potential complications may be quite serious.

## What Are the Symptoms?

The symptoms, causes, and possible complications of urinary tract infections depend on the age of the child. Generally, the younger the child, the less specific the symptoms are. Symptoms of a UTI in older children and adults include pain on urination, frequent urination, and new onset of bedwetting. Other less frequent symptoms include blood in the urine, abdominal pain, and sometimes a low-grade fever. Symptoms indicative of a kidney infection, known as pyelonephritis, are back pain, high fever, chills, and sometimes vomiting. In younger children and babies, the symptoms are even less specific and may include only fever, increased irritability, decreased feeding, diarrhea, and/or vomiting.

## What Tests Can Confirm a Urinary Infection?

The only way to determine whether or not a child has a UTI is to do a urine test. Collecting urine from a baby is a challenge. A commonly used technique is to attach a plastic bag around a child's genitalia and wait until the child voids into the bag so that the urine can be analyzed. Another way of obtaining urine is by a catheter—a small tube inserted into the child's urethra. Once collected, the urine is analyzed and examined microscopically in order to confirm the presence of infection.

The definitive test to confirm a UTI, however, is to send the urine for culturing. This takes twenty-four to forty-eight hours and confirms or denies the presence of a bacterial infection in the urine.

## How Are Urinary Infections Treated?

The treatment for a UTI is antibiotics. Which one, how it is administered, and for how long depends on the age and history of the child, as well as on how sick a child with a suspected UTI looks. Certainly in young or sick-looking children, healthcare providers will not wait twenty-four to forty-eight hours for the culture results before starting treatment. If the initial analysis is abnormal and suggestive of a UTI, treatment will be started before the culture results come out. In young babies, children who are vomiting, and children with a suspected kidney infection, antibiotics are given intravenously in hospital. Usually, older children who are not sick looking and have no obvious complications are treated with antibiotics given by mouth.

## Are Other Test Needed?

The other issues in children with a UTI are possible underlying kidney or bladder abnormalities. It is for this reason that most young children with a UTI, especially boys, need special tests to ensure that there are no kidney or bladder problems. Typically a kidney ultrasound is performed, which can tell us about the kidney, bladder, and urinary system in general.

If the ultrasound reading is not normal, depending on the results and the specific situation, another test may be needed. It is called a voiding cystourethrogram (VCUG). This test determines whether the connection between the kidneys and the bladder—the ureters—work well or not. If there is an abnormality detected, this means that children will be prone to getting repeat infections. The treatment of these anomalies, such as abnormally shaped kidneys, an abnormal collecting system, and a urinary flow known as vesicoureteral reflux, ranges from taking preventative antibiotics daily to an operation to repair the congenital abnormality. In certain situations other tests may also be necessary to assess how the kidneys are working and to what degree they may be blocked.

# West Nile Virus

West Nile virus belongs to a family of viruses called *Flaviviridae* and was first isolated in 1937 in the West Nile sub-region of Uganda. The first West Nile virus infection in North America occurred in New York City in the summer of 1999. In Canada, the virus was first found in birds in Ontario in 2001.

## How Do People Get Infected With West Nile Virus?

Most people infected with West Nile virus got it from the bite of an infected mosquito. A mosquito becomes infected when it feeds on a bird that is infected with the virus. The mosquito can then pass the virus to people and animals by biting them. Probably less than 1 percent of mosquitoes in any given area are infected with West Nile virus. This means the risk of being bitten by an infected mosquito is low. But, it could happen to anyone in areas where West Nile virus is active.

There have been cases of West Nile virus spreading through blood transfusions and organ transplants. However, there is no evidence to suggest that people can get West Nile virus by touching or kissing someone who is infected, or from being around a healthcare worker who has treated an infected person. There is no evidence that the virus can pass directly from infected animals (horses, pets, etcetera) to people.

## Who Is Most at Risk?

Many people infected with West Nile virus have mild symptoms or no symptoms at all. Although anybody can have serious health effects, it is people with weaker immune systems who are at greater risk for serious complications. This higher risk group includes the following:

- People over the age of forty;
- People with chronic diseases, such as cancer, diabetes, and heart disease;
- People who require medical treatment or medications that may weaken their immune system (such as chemotherapy or corticosteroids).

Although individuals with weaker immune systems are at greater risk, West Nile virus can cause severe complications for people of any age and any health status. This is why it is so important to reduce the risk of getting bitten by mosquitoes.

## The Symptoms of West Nile Virus Infection

Symptoms usually appear within two to fifteen days. The type and severity of symptoms vary from person to person.

Symptoms of mild disease include the following:

- Flu-like symptoms;
- Fever;
- Headache;
- Body aches;
- Rash.

Persons with weaker immune systems or a chronic disease are at greater risk of developing more serious complications, including meningitis (infection of the covering of the brain) and encephalitis (infection of the brain itself). Tragically, these conditions can be fatal.

Symptoms of more severe disease include the following:

- Severe headache;
- High fever;
- Stiff neck;
- Nausea and vomiting;
- Sleepiness;
- Confusion;
- Loss of consciousness;
- Lack of coordination;
- Muscle weakness and paralysis.

## Is There a Treatment for West Nile Virus Infection?

Unfortunately, as with most viruses, there is no specific treatment or medication for West Nile virus. Serious cases receive supportive treatments, such as intravenous fluids, close monitoring, and medications that help fight the complications of the infection. Obviously, such cases may require hospitalization. Currently, there is no vaccine available to protect against West Nile virus, although there is a lot of research going on in this area.

## How Is West Nile Virus Infection Confirmed?

If a healthcare provider suspects that a person may have West Nile virus, based on the history of symptoms, especially in an area where West Nile virus is present, there are specific blood tests that can confirm the infection.

## Mosquito Bite Prevention

The best way to reduce the risk of infection is to try to prevent mosquito bites. See the suggestions given in the safety section at the front of this book.

# Whooping Cough

Infants and young children are routinely vaccinated against whooping cough (also known as pertussis). However, we are still seeing cases of whooping cough in babies and young adults. Because the vaccine seems to wear off, older adults get infected with mild symptoms and unknowingly pass it on to babies who are not yet fully protected.

Whooping cough is caused by a bacterium called *Bordetella Pertussis*, which is spread through the air when an infected person coughs. Whooping cough tends to spread more easily in close-contact situations, such as among family members and in schools. The infection begins like a regular cold and then the very characteristic cough phase develops. The cough occurs in spurts during which a person's face turns red, their eyes become teary, and they often vomit after the cough. There is a very characteristic whooping sound during the cough, giving the very scary impression of choking. This cough phase can last for up to three months and typically slowly goes away on its own. Although it causes great discomfort, pertussis is not considered life-threatening in older children and healthy adults. However, it can be very dangerous, even deadly, in infants and young babies.

## Whooping Cough Treatment

Unfortunately, antibiotics do not usually change the duration of the symptoms. Antibiotics are generally given to the individual and close contacts to stop the spread of the bacteria. The only available treatment is supportive, including cough medicines, depending on the age and circumstances, which are given only under the direct supervision of a healthcare provider. Babies with whooping cough are usually hospitalized for very close monitoring and support.

## Whooping Cough Prevention

The pertussis vaccine has been very helpful in preventing whooping cough over the last several decades. However, the older pertussis vaccine was not 100 percent effective; it wore off with age and had some potentially serious side effects. It was initially given five times, incorporated with the routine vaccine schedule with the last booster given between four and six years of age.

A newer version was developed, known as the Acellular pertussis vaccine, combined with the diphtheria-tetanus vaccine, which was given six times, the last dose being during the teenage years, around the ages of fourteen and fifteen. More recently, we have noticed that, despite vaccinating teenagers with the extra booster shot, we still see cases among babies. For this reason, this vaccine is now available to adults between sixteen and sixty-four years of age who have not received their sixth shot. This one-time extra dose will hopefully boost adults' immunity and indirectly, surrounding children (be it their kids, the neighbors' kids, grandkids, nephews, and nieces etcetera).

Administering a booster dose of the Acellular pertussis vaccine to adults will make a difference in the rates of this infection among younger children. All adults may talk with their healthcare provider or local public health agency about this shot, especially if they are in contact with young infants and babies.

# Index

N



O



P



R



S



T



U

## Author Biography

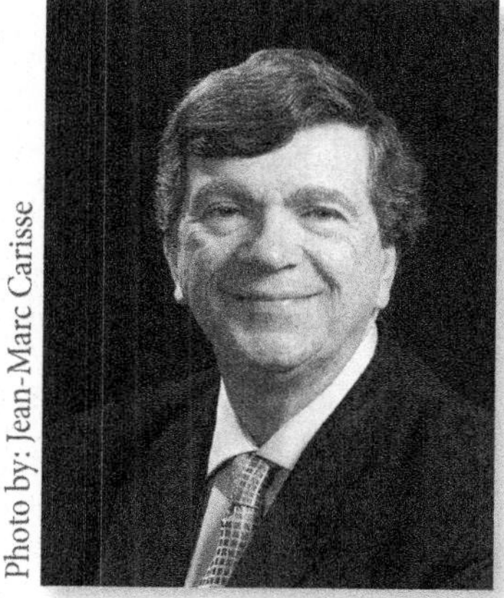
Photo by: Jean-Marc Carisse

Pediatrician DR.PAUL Roumeliotis is a true health communications pioneer. Over the last two decades, he has educated millions worldwide through his ground-breaking website, audio cassettes, videos, and DVDs. DR.PAUL is also featured regularly on TV (CTV-2) and for many years on his radio segments and shows.

Certified by the American Board of Pediatrics and the Royal College of Physicians of Canada, DR.PAUL is the founder and former director of the Montreal Children's Hospital Pediatric Consultation and Asthma Centres. He is an adjunct professor of pediatrics and former director of Multi-Format Health Communications for the Faculty of Medicine at McGill University in Montreal, Canada. He also holds a Masters of Public Health degree from Johns Hopkins University Bloomberg School of Public Health where he is an Associate faculty member. His specific interest and focus is on early child development support and its effects over the course of a lifetime.

# DR. PAUL'S INFORMATION

A health communications pioneer and pediatrician, DR.PAUL Roumeliotis believes that the future of healthcare is in communicating health information in a variety of media formats, thereby making it available to the largest audience possible. It was this vision that inspired him to become a writer/publisher/producer of multi-format health and wellness resources, including becoming the world's first online pediatrician with a website that has been visited by millions since its launch in 1995.

Beginning as a professional drummer and record producer, DR. PAUL's journey to his present vision actually preceded his medical career. In 1991, he merged his medical expertise and technical talents into the ***DR. PAUL Child Health and Wellness Information Project***, reflecting his commitment to create practical and trustworthy health information resources in all formats. He has created and produced well over 300 productions (more than 1 million of his videos, cassettes, and DVDs have been distributed across North America) including:

- *Welcoming Baby Home* Video: distributed for free across Canada
- *Wellness for Mothers to Be* Video and Booklet: distributed for free across Canada
- *Best For Baby: A Healthy First Year* Video: distributed for free across Canada
- *Understanding Ear Infections, A Video Guide for Parents*: distributed for free across Canada

DR.PAUL has been able to effectively merge his skills in producing information with accuracy, credibility, confidence, and comfort as a common theme. The potential social impact is enormous, as the need for accurate and empathetic health content is huge.

**DR.PAUL's first published book, *Baby Comes Home*, which focuses on early child development support and its effects over the course of a lifetime, is another of his numerous health educational projects for families and child caregivers worldwide.**

For more information, please visit: **www.drpaul.com**

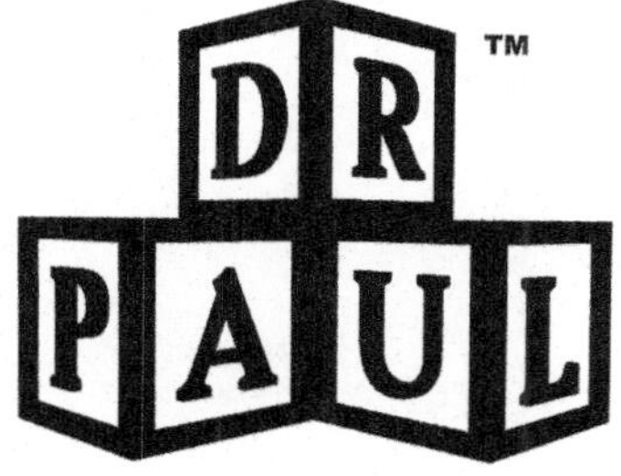

If you want to get on the path to be a published author by Influence Publishing please go to www.InfluencePublishing.com

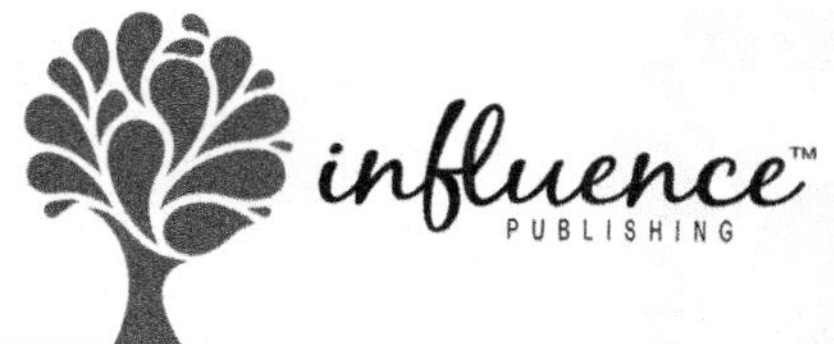


More information on our other titles and how to submit your own proposal can be found at www.InfluencePublishing.com

CPSIA information can be obtained at www.ICGtesting.com
Printed in the USA
LVOW04s1745061214

417537LV00001B/1/P

9 781771 410724